T0269269

Case Studies in Sports Psychiatry

A fascinating, accessible and much needed guide to this important and emerging sub-speciality. This book feels fresh, relevant and gives an in-depth understanding while providing the reader with the tools they need to really get to grips with the subject. This book is a trailblazer, and destined to become a definitive classic in the area. I hate sport and even I loved this book.

Dr Max Pemberton, Psychiatrist and Daily Mail Columnist

Case Studies in Sports Psychiatry has several unique features that make it an invaluable resource for those interested in the rapidly evolving field of athlete mental health. The comprehensive yet concise case studies provide practical insight into the presentation, assessment and management of common mental health problems across a variety of high-profile sports. Readers benefit from authorship by expert practitioners working at the athlete health front-line, with the detailed answers to the questions tabled at the end of each chapter demonstrating that effective mental health support requires an inter-disciplinary approach – making this a book for everyone involved in athlete care.

Dr Craig Ranson, Director of Athlete, English Institute of Sport

Case Studies in Sports Psychiatry is a must-read for those who care for the mental health of elite athletes. The authors make a substantial thought provoking contribution to the science of how psychiatric support can be provided to athletes who experience mental illness. Authors achieve this through comprehensive case reviews of athletes from various sports, levels of performance, ages, and genders. This book is the first of its kind with a focus on mental illness, and I have no doubt it will make an excellent contribution to psychiatry training, as well as trigger interest from colleagues in Sports Medicine, Sport and Exercise Psychology, sport science and coaching. The book contributes to increasing knowledge of the dangers of mental health stigma in sport culture and will inevitably contribute to training Sport Psychiatrists, which in turn will improve the lives of our elite sports people.

Dr Gavin Breslin, Senior Lecturer in Sport and Exercise Psychology,
School of Psychology, Ulster University, Northern Ireland and Chief
Assessor for the Qualification in Sport and Exercise Psychology,
British Psychological Society

An informative, enlightening and attention grabbing read in an emerging field where the evidence base is developing fast. The use of real-life scenarios developed from the lived experience of athletes brings the subject alive is educationally stimulating.

We like to think that athletes are superhuman, but they struggle and become ill like the rest of us. Fortunately effective, evidence-based treatments are available. The editors and contributors are at the forefront of this endeavour and have thankfully shared their knowledge and expertise in this book. The causes and presentation of mental illness in athletes brings unique challenges and treatments are often constrained by the complex environments inhabited by elite sports people.

The reader is taken on a journey accompanied by the athlete and clinician and is led through examples of how mental illness presents and invited by means of probing questions to engage in the exploration of care and treatment. I thoroughly recommend this book to all those engaged with the mental health of athletes but to psychiatrists generally and to all those interested in sports science.

Dr Adrian James, President, Royal College of Psychiatrists

Case Studies in Sports Psychiatry

Edited by

Amit D Mistry
Barnet, Enfield and Haringey Mental Health NHS Trust

Thomas McCabe
NHS Greater Glasgow and Clyde

Alan Currie
Cumbria, Northumberland, Tyne and Wear NHS Foundation Trust

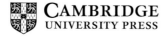

CAMBRIDGE
UNIVERSITY PRESS

CAMBRIDGE
UNIVERSITY PRESS

University Printing House, Cambridge CB2 8BS, United Kingdom

One Liberty Plaza, 20th Floor, New York, NY 10006, USA

477 Williamstown Road, Port Melbourne, VIC 3207, Australia

314–321, 3rd Floor, Plot 3, Splendor Forum, Jasola District Centre,
New Delhi – 110025, India

79 Anson Road, #06–04/06, Singapore 079906

Cambridge University Press is part of the University of Cambridge.

It furthers the University's mission by disseminating knowledge in the pursuit of
education, learning, and research at the highest international levels of excellence.

www.cambridge.org
Information on this title: www.cambridge.org/9781108720557
DOI: 10.1017/9781108767187

First published 2020

A catalogue record for this publication is available from the British Library.

Library of Congress Cataloging-in-Publication Data
Names: Mistry, Amit D., editor. | McCabe, Thomas (Psychiatrist), editor. | Currie, Alan, editor.
Title: Case studies in sports psychiatry / edited by Amit D. Mistry, University College London, Thomas
McCabe, West of Scotland Deanery, Alan Currie, Northumberland, Tyne and West NHS Foundation Trust.
Description: Cambridge, United Kingdom ; New York, NY : Cambridge University Press, 2020. | Includes
bibliographical references and index.
Identifiers: LCCN 2020011455 | ISBN 9781108720557 (paperback) | ISBN 9781108767187 (ebook)
Subjects: LCSH: Athletes – Mental health – Case studies.
Classification: LCC RC451.4.A83 C37 2020 | DDC 616.890088/796–dc23
LC record available at https://lccn.loc.gov/2020011455

ISBN 978-1-108-72055-7 Paperback

Contents

Editors

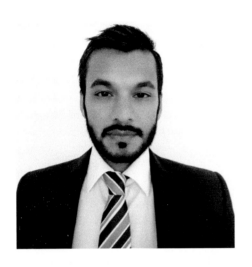

Amit D Mistry (@DrAMistryPsych)

General Adult and Old Age Psychiatrist, IANLP, BSc, MB ChB, MRCPsych

Dr Amit D Mistry is dual trained in general adult and old age psychiatry based in north London and Chair of the Royal College of Psychiatrists' (RCPsych) Sports and Exercise Psychiatry Special Interest Group (SEPSIG). He is an honorary clinical lecturer in Sports and Exercise Medicine (SEM) at the Queen Mary University of London.

His published research is related to exercise, exercise addiction, eating disorders and wellbeing within the sport, leisure and fitness industry. He is an expert panel member for Mind charity's physical activity programme and is on the NHS clinical entrepreneurship programme. Amit is an ex-county rugby union player and represented Team GB at the International Rugby Tag Federation World Cup.

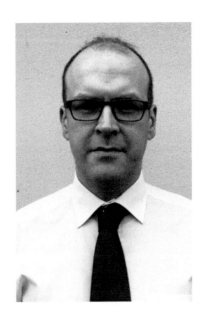

Thomas McCabe (@Dr_t_mccabe)

Old Age Psychiatrist, MB ChB, MRCPsych

Dr Thomas McCabe is a psychiatrist based in Glasgow. Following graduating from the University of Aberdeen, he initially trained in general practice before choosing psychiatry as a career and was shortlisted for Royal College of Psychiatry trainee of the year in 2017. Dr McCabe has published articles in various leading journals including the British Journal of Sports Medicine on mental health and sport. He is an honorary clinical lecturer at the University of Glasgow. Dr McCabe is a researcher and author with the landmark FIELD study (Football's InfluencE on Lifelong health and Dementia risk). He has presented at national events on the topic and plays a central role in the Royal College of Psychiatrists' SEPSIG with particular interest in students and trainee psychiatrists. Dr McCabe was the first psychiatrist to devise a mental health strategy for an elite level football team. Dr McCabe also has psychiatric expertise in rugby, cricket, suicidality in athletes and longer-term cognitive outcomes in contact sport athletes.

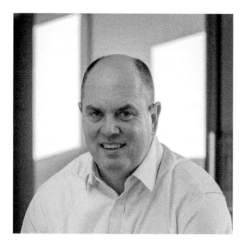

Alan Currie

Consultant Psychiatrist, MB ChB, MPhil, FRCPsych

Professor Alan Currie is a consultant psychiatrist in Newcastle and a visiting professor at the University of Sunderland in the department of sport and exercise sciences. His research interests include recovery, social inclusion, mood disorders, movement disorders and sport and exercise psychiatry. He has published in all these areas and edited a highly commended handbook of sports psychiatry in 2016.

He was founder and inaugural chair of SEPSIG of the Royal College of Psychiatrists and a member of the International Society for Sports Psychiatry (ISSP). He joined the International Olympic Committee mental health working group in 2018. In 2019, he was appointed to the Mental Health Expert Panel of the English Institute of Sport (EIS).

Contributors

Dr Marwan Al-Dawoud is a sport and exercise medicine physician and primary care physician based in West Yorkshire. He has worked in elite sport since 2007 across rugby league, rugby union, football, athletics and ballet at national and international levels. He is heavily involved across NHS musculoskeletal services across the United Kingdom. He is a reviewer for the *British Medical Journal* and is actively involved in research and education.

Dr Richard Budgett has been medical and scientific director of the International Olympic Committee (IOC) since November 2012. Before that he was chief medical officer for the London 2012 Olympic and Paralympic Games from 2007 to 2012. He was director of medical services for the British Olympic Association from 1994 to 2007 and has been chief medical officer with Team GB at the summer and winter Olympic Games in Atlanta, Nagano, Sydney, Salt Lake City, Athens and Turin. He won an Olympic Gold medal in rowing in the Olympic Games Los Angeles 1984.

Naomi Cavaday is a former professional British tennis player whose highest British Women's ranking was that of number three. She has won individual International Tennis Federation titles and has performed coaching roles with the Lawn Tennis Association (LTA). Naomi remains a mental health ambassador for British tennis, co-hosts the @tennispodcast1 podcast and commentates for BBC Radio 5 Live's Wimbledon coverage.

Dr Robin Chatterjee is a consultant in sports and exercise medicine. He is the lead academy doctor at West Ham United Football Club; medical officer at London Broncos Rugby Football League Club; co-founder of Panacea Health and works at St George's NHS Foundation Trust.

David Cotterill is an ex-international, Welsh professional footballer and has gained 20 international caps for this country. He started his footballing career at Bristol City and made his Premier League debut for Wigan Athletic in 2006. He has played for other high-profile clubs and is now a proud ambassador for mental health and addictions awareness within professional football.

Dr Shane Creado is a sports psychiatrist, and is double board-certified in psychiatry and sleep medicine. He is a published author, and focuses on sleep optimisation in elite athletes, integrative psychiatry and brain SPECT imaging. He has been on the board of directors of the ISSP, as its chairman of memberships and mentoring.

Dr James Dove is a general adult psychiatrist working in north London. He is in his final year of higher training and is pursuing a career as a consultant liaison psychiatrist. In 2018, he completed his postgraduate certificate in leadership in health (Darzi Fellowship) at London Southbank University, sponsored by Camden and Islington NHS Foundation Trust.

Dr Emily Dudgeon competed over 800m, coming 6th at the World Juniors in 2012 and narrowly missing out on the final of the Commonwealth Games in 2014. Since then, she has qualified as a doctor and is passionate about raising awareness of RED-S and eating disorders in sport, having seen these issues affect the athletic potential, mental and physical health of friends in the sport.

Patrick Foster is a former professional cricketer whose life was torn to shreds by his pathological gambling addiction. Patrick's life became monopolised by gambling from his university days onwards as he found making the transition from playing sport and into the real world a huge challenge. He is now the head of education at EPIC risk management, leading harm-minimisation and awareness experts related to gambling and gaming addiction.

Dr Phil Hopley is a former London Wasps semi-professional rugby player who also represented England students and the Barbarians in the 1990s. He is a Consultant Psychiatrist and MD at Cognacity where he runs the Sport Mental Health team looking after 15 UK individual and team sports. In 2012, Phil ran the Cognacity Mental Health Team covering the 10,000 athletes at the London Olympic and Paralympic Games.

Marsha Hull is a professional golfer and a Professional Golfers' Association (PGA) teacher. She has supported medical services for the European Tour Performance Institute and has caddied on professional tours.

Dr Allan Johnston is a consultant psychiatrist specialising in sports psychiatry via Synergy Medicine Ltd, an independent sports medicine service in Leeds. He is the current finance officer for the Royal College of Psychiatrists' SEPSIG. Dr Johnston is employed by the EIS as sports psychiatrist to the mental health expert panel supporting Great Britain Olympic and Paralympic athletes in preparation for the Tokyo Olympic Games in 2020. Also, he works as a consultant performance psychiatrist to the League Managers Association in a role to guide and shape the mental health and

wellbeing programme for Premier League and football league managers.

Joe Kasper is a US-based American football coach and currently works with Duke University's team. He has previously worked with National Football League (NFL) outfits such as the Cleveland Browns and has former collegiate-level playing experience with Baldwin Wallace University.

Dr Simon Kemp is a specialist in sports and exercise medicine and the medical services director of the Rugby Football Union, responsible for their clinical services, player welfare, anti-doping and research functions across the elite, community and age-group games.

Dr Jo Larkin is a consultant in sports and exercise medicine. She is the current chief medical officer for the LTA and works with British elite tennis players and future aspiring junior players. She has worked in military medicine and been involved with two Olympic Games and one Paralympic Games.

Dr Catherine Lester is a sports and exercise medicine consultant. She is the team doctor for Northampton Saints Rugby Football Club and works in private practice. Also, Catherine works with Moving Medicine©, an initiative designed to promote physical activity for both medical and mental health conditions.

Dr Hassan Mahmood is a consultant psychiatrist based in Birmingham. He has a special interest in the mental health of sportsmen, particularly elite cricketers.

Renee McGregor is a leading sports and eating disorder specialist dietitian with 20 years' experience working in clinical and performance nutrition. She is the co-founder of #TRAINBRAVE, one of the most successful campaigns raising the awareness of eating disorders in sport and dance. She is on the RED-S advisory board for the British Association of Sport and Exercise Science and sits on the international task force for orthorexia.

Adrian Moorhouse is a former Olympic swimmer who won Gold in the 100m breaststroke at the Seoul Olympic Games in 1988. He co-founded performance consultancy Lane4 in 1995, which uses insight from business, psychology and elite sport to help businesses develop their people skills to become winning organisations.

Dr Andrew Murray is chief medical officer of the PGA European Tour, responsible for its worldwide medical operations, its advisory board and the research programme. He is a member of the medical commission of the International Golf Federation. His PhD funded by the World Golf Foundation looks at golf and health.

Dr Caz Nahman is a child and adolescent psychiatrist specialising in eating disorders and has an interest in athletes, compulsive exercise and eating disorders. She is a previous executive committee member of the Royal College of Psychiatrist's Eating Disorders faculty and is co-editor of the book *New to Eating Disorders* (Cambridge University Press).

Dr Mayur Pandya is a US board-certified psychiatrist with expertise working with elite athletes and professional sports organisations in the National Basketball Association, Major League Baseball, NFL/NFL Players Association and collegiate athletics. He completed his psychiatry residency training at Cleveland Clinic and is the director of ACE Sports Psychiatry in Cleveland, Ohio (US).

Cyrus Pattinson is a Northumberland boxer representing Team GB with aspirations to compete at the Tokyo 2020 Olympic Games before pursuing a professional career. Alongside his boxing career, Cyrus is a strong mental health advocate.

Professor Steve Peters is a UK-based psychiatrist who has worked in elite sport covering over 20 national teams and has attended four Olympic Games. He has acted as an expert witness to the World Anti-Doping Agency (WADA) and was a member of the UK Therapeutic Use Exemption (TUE) panel for over a decade. As an author, he has published the highly acclaimed book *The Chimp Paradox*.

Dr Carolyn Plateau is based at Loughborough University as a lecturer in psychology. Carolyn's area of research expertise is focused around understanding the risks and consequences of disordered eating and exercise among athletes. Her research has led to the development of screening tools, educational materials and resources to support sports professionals in the prevention, identification and management of disordered eating among athletes.

Dr Rebecca Robinson is a consultant in sports and exercise medicine, working with elite and amateur athletes to optimise mental and physical health. She possesses a special interest in managing aspects of relative energy deficiency that can impact both athletes' wellbeing and performance and crucially longer-term health.

Dr Tim Rogers is a consultant sports psychiatrist and applied sport and exercise psychology graduate working at Cognacity, London. Tim sits on the Sport Resolutions National Anti-Doping Panel and is an executive member of the Royal College of Psychiatrists' SEPSIG. In 2019, Dr Rogers was appointed clinical director of Big White Wall, the UK's leading digital mental health service, which provides a service to all UK

Sport/EIS coaches and athletes competing at the Tokyo 2020 Olympic Games.

Luke Rowe is a professional Welsh cyclist for Team Ineos and has been with them for over seven years. He has been part of the winning Tour de France squad for the last four seasons, specialises in classic cycling and is considered a rouleur within his field.

Steve Sanders is a former professional NFL player and has played for the Cleveland Browns, Detroit Lions and Arizona Cardinals. Since retiring from the NFL in 2012, he has published *Training Camp For Life: Developing Champions In Sports and In Life* and has worked as an ambassador for the NFL college outreach programme. During the NFL season he hosts a weekly TV Show *Straight From The Pros* on NBC-WKYC as the on-air sports analyst.

Dr Willie Stewart is a consultant neuro-pathologist at the Queen Elizabeth University Hospital, Glasgow, and holds honorary associate professor status at the universities of Glasgow (Institute of Neuroscience and Psychology) and Pennsylvania (Department of Neurosurgery). He leads an internationally regarded research laboratory engaged in multiple programmes investigating the pathologies of acute and long-term survival from sports-related head injury. Also, Dr Stewart directs the FIELD study, which aims to describe lifelong health and dementia risk in former soccer players.

Rob Vickerman is a former professional English rugby union player and ex-captain of the England rugby sevens team. Following retirement he has worked as a broadcaster for various channels such as the BBC, Radio 5 Live, Channel 5, Sky Sports and World Rugby. Rob regularly commentates on both the rugby sevens and fifteens games. He has covered events such as the Rugby World Cup (2015 and 2019), Olympic Games (Rio, 2016) and the rugby sevens world series. Also, he is the founder of Work Athlete UK, an organisation that focuses on employee performance and productivity within the workplace.

Foreword

Mental health disorders are common in elite athletes and mental health is now recognised as a crucial component of athlete health, relating closely to both physical health and performance. Mental health symptoms and disorders increase the risk of injury and delay recovery of athletes.

Those caring for the athlete (the athlete entourage) are often poorly educated in the diagnosis and management of mental health disorders, which frequently present in a complex and atypical manner in athletes compared to the general population. Those caring for athletes need to differentiate character traits unique to elite athletes from psychosocial maladaptation and then need to consider the unique biopsychosocial factors relevant to athletes in order to address all the factors contributing to mental health symptoms. The environment in which athletes compete and train needs to be assessed and managed, as well as treating the individual athlete appropriately using mental health tools and specialist help where needed. The realisation of these important challenges in the prevention, diagnosis and management of elite athletes led to the IOC holding a consensus meeting on athlete mental health in 2018 which led to the publication of the 2019 IOC consensus statement on mental health disorders in elite athletes along with sub-specialty papers, and a toolkit for athletes and their entourage based on the consensus.

Internationally, no published book has focused on athlete mental health issues using in-depth case-based discussions. This textbook takes a novel approach through in-depth case studies, and is designed to map onto the latest ISSP educational curriculum. Each chapter focuses on an elite/professional athlete with a mental health condition that is relevant to their sporting discipline. In addition, reader knowledge is assessed through Multiple Choice Questionnaires and True or False questions.

This academic book also educates allied sports healthcare professionals on how sports psychiatrists can help athletes experiencing psychiatric morbidity. It will help readers gain a better understanding of the unique risk factors, and identification and manifestations of psychiatric disorders within each sporting discipline. It also outlines potential ethical challenges in patient care and how to provide evidence-based, tailored psychiatric support incorporating holistic, biopsychosocial principles.

This textbook of sports psychiatry is a useful resource for all members of the multidisciplinary team caring for athletes who are interested in mental health as well as psychiatrists wishing to venture into this exciting, growing field. The book is aimed at all healthcare professionals in the field of sports and exercise medicine particularly consultants in sports and exercise medicine, team doctors, psychiatrists and psychologists. It should be a useful resource for key allied healthcare professionals, coaches, career advisors and counsellors involved in elite sport, too.

The editors are executive members of the Royal College of Psychiatrist's SEPSIG group and ISSP. Chapter co-authors include sports psychiatrists, sports and exercise medicine clinicians, allied health professionals and former professional/elite athletes.

There have been welcome developments in recent years to reduce the stigma attached to mental health problems in sport and improve the support that athletes receive. This textbook will contribute to continued progress in mental health treatment and care in the world of sport.

Richard Budgett
OBE MA MBBS FRCP FFSEM FISM Dip Sports Med

Preface

Amit Mistry, Thomas McCabe and Alan Currie

Scepticism of psychiatry's place in the world of sport was clearly articulated in Dan Begel's 1992 description of the foundations and framework of sports psychiatry practice (1). Since then the move to acceptance has been gradual and perhaps begins with the establishment of the International Society for Sports Psychiatry (ISSP) in 1994. Twenty-five years later there is widespread acknowledgement of the mental health symptoms and disorders that can develop in sport as evidenced by the IOC's consensus statement on athlete mental health (2) and an entire issue of the *British Journal of Sports Medicine* devoted to mental health in June 2019. There have also been a series of theory- and practice-based textbooks and manuals including *Sport Psychiatry* (3), *Sports Psychiatry: Strategies for Life Balance and Peak Performance* (4), *Clinical Sports Psychiatry* (5), a *Sports Psychiatry* handbook (6) and *The ISSP Manual of Sports Psychiatry* (7). A curriculum has been developed by the ISSP to support training in sports psychiatry and the role of the psychiatrist in the assessment, treatment and rehabilitation of athletes with mental health problems has been described (8). Despite this there is a paucity of sports-specific research on treatments (9,10,11), clinicians must extrapolate from treatment evidence in general populations and practise thoughtful and safe 'individualised prescribing' (12) and clinical opinion still exceeds experimental evidence (13).

Athletes experience mental health problems through a combination of generic and sports-specific factors (2,9). Indeed, 640 different stressors have been described across all sports (14) although the key stressors would appear to be musculoskeletal problems, frequent surgeries, problems with sporting performance and maladaptive perfectionism (2). Coincidence may also be a factor with the peak age of sporting performance coinciding with the age of onset of conditions such as bipolar and psychotic disorders (15,16). Although mental health problems may be as common in sporting populations as in the general population (and in some cases more common) (17) their presentation may be unusual when the disorder emerges in the world of sport (17), and diagnosing anxiety disorders, eating disorders, depression and hypomania may pose special problems in the world of high-performance sport (18). Psychiatric care is 'often delivered without a full understanding of the diagnostic and therapeutic issues unique to this population' (10).

To deliver good psychiatric treatment and care to athletes requires an approach that is comprehensive, integrative and athlete centred (2). Emotional, physical, social and environmental factors need consideration (2) and the biopsychosocial model that prevails in psychiatric practice lends itself to this (8). Clinicians who work in sport need to be flexible to accommodate the busy schedules of sportsmen and women (19) and reach out to them (8,20) yet not succumb to vicarious gratification in counter-transference (1,21) by offering special treatment to the elite athlete (19). The practice of a sports psychiatrist will also include taking a comprehensive sport and exercise history (20) alongside a more traditional personal and developmental history and is likely to require working with the athlete's coach and others in the support team who are key members of the athlete's 'surrogate family' (20). Like other practitioners who work in sport the psychiatrist will undertake an assessment process and develop a treatment plan that understands not only the nature of the illness or condition but also the affected individual and the context or environment in which disorder has developed.

Psychiatric practice in the sporting environment has limited specific evidence on which to base treatment and therapy. Clinicians must use existing evidence from general populations and apply this in an unusual and often extreme set of circumstances. It is for these reasons that we have collected a series of case studies to illustrate the range of mental health problems and disorders that present in sport and to guide the clinician in ways of approaching assessment and treatment in support of the athlete's health and performance. Following case-study learning theory we have strived to demonstrate how psychiatric consultations can be structured and review some of the latest evidence base for managing mental illness within different sporting disciplines. Sports psychiatry is still in its relative infancy and as the evidence base continues to grow, we hope over time to provide more definitive guidance on how to recognise and treat mental health problems within the elite sport setting. Currently, proposed treatment plans may vary dependent on a psychiatrist's own clinical expertise with different assessment tools, psychotropic medication and psychotherapeutic treatment modalities. Despite this potential variance in practice, all agreed plans should follow a patient-centred, comprehensive biopsychosocial approach.

At the first consultation, patients may be reluctant to disclose sensitive personal information and the clinician may have a limited time frame to complete the initial assessment. Therefore, a diagnostic formulation is unlikely to be through following a one-off consultation, particularly as the clinician–patient therapeutic relationship takes time to develop. Also, insights from alternative information sources such as family and team members and previous mental health records will add to the developing understanding of the athlete's problems and predicament. We also acknowledge that for all mental health conditions there is not a single 'right answer' nor even universality of approach. By using case studies we aim to illustrate common clinical problems and suggested management but recognise that experienced clinicians bring their own wisdom and a variety of management strategies to each individual patient.

The project has been a joint endeavour between experts from many disciplines and athletes who are experts by experience. We aim to raise awareness and create stigma-free, parity of esteem for mental health treatment in the elite sport setting and we hope this book will also stimulate the reader to research and learn more about sports psychiatry.

References

1. Begel D. An overview of sport psychiatry. *Am J Psychiatry*. 1992;149(5)(May):606–14.

2. Reardon CL, Hainline B, Aron CM, Baron D, Baum AL, Bindra A, et al. Mental health in elite athletes: International Olympic Committee consensus statement (2019). *Br J Sports Med*. 2019 [cited 2019 May 29];53 (11):667–99. Available from: www.ncbi.nlm.nih.gov/pubmed/31097450

3. Begel D, Burton RW. *Sport Psychiatry*. Begel D, Burton RW, eds. New York: WW Norton; 2000 [cited 2016 Feb 15]. Available from: http://books.wwnorton.com/books/Sport-Psychiatry/

4. McDuff DR. *Sports Psychiatry: Strategies for Life Balance and Peak Performance*. Washington, DC. American Psychiatric Publishing, Inc. 2012.

5. Baron DA, Reardon CL, Baron SH, eds. *Clinical Sports Psychiatry: An International Perspective*. New York. John Wiley and Sons. 2013.

6. Currie A, Owen B. *Sports Psychiatry*. Currie A, Owen B, eds. Oxford University Press; 2016 [cited 2016 Apr 30]. Available from: www.oxfordmedicine.com/view/10.1093/med/9780198734628.001.0001/med-9780198734628

7. Glick ID, Kamis D, Stull T, eds.*The ISSP Manual of Sports Psychiatry*. 1st edition. New York: Routledge; 2018.

8. Currie A, Johnston A. Psychiatric disorders: The psychiatrist's contribution to sport. *Int Rev Psychiatry* . 2016 [cited 2016 Dec 7];28(6):587–94. Available from: www.tandfonline.com/doi/full/10.1080/09540261.2016.1197188

9. Rice SM, Purcell R, De Silva S, Mawren D, McGorry PD, Parker AG. The mental health of elite athletes: A narrative systematic review. *Sport Med*. 2016;46 (9):1333–53. Available from: http://dx.doi .org/10.1007/s40279-016-0492-2

10. Reardon CL, Factor RM. Sport Psychiatry: A systematic review of diagnosis and medical treatment of mental illness in athletes. *Sport Med*. 2010;40(11):961–80. Available from: http://ovidsp.ovid.com/ov idweb.cgi?T=JS&PAGE=reference&D=me d5&NEWS=N&AN=20942511%5Cnhtt p://link.springer.com/10.2165/11536580-0 00000000-00000

11. Reardon CL. The sports psychiatrist and psychiatric medication. *Int Rev Psychiatry*. 2016 [cited 2016 Dec 7];28(6):606–13. Available from: www.tandfonline.com/doi/full/10.1080/09540261.2016.1190691

12. Johnston A, McAllister-Williams RH. Psychotropic Drug Prescribing. In: Currie A, Owen B, eds. *Sports Psychiatry*. 1st edition. Oxford. Oxford University Press. 2016. p. 133–43.

13. Begel D. Sport psychiatry twenty-four years later. *Int Rev Psychiatry* . 2016; 1–4. Available from: www.tandfonline.com/doi/full/10.1080/09540261.2016.1202215

14. Arnold R, Fletcher D. A research synthesis and taxonomic classification of the organizational stressors encountered by sport performers. *J Sport Exerc Psychol*. 2012 [cited 2019 Jun 14];34(3):397–429.

Available from: http://journals.humanki netics.com/doi/10.1123/jsep.34.3.397

15. Moesch K, Kenttä G, Kleinert J, Quignon-Fleuret C, Cecil S, Bertollo M. FEPSAC position statement: Mental health disorders in elite athletes and models of service provision. *Psychol Sport Exerc*. 2018;(38):61–71. Available from: www.sci encedirect.com/science/article/pii/ S1469029218300153

16. Currie A, Gorczynski P, Rice SM, Purcell R, McAllister-Williams RH, Hitchcock ME, et al. Bipolar and psychotic disorders in elite athletes: a narrative review. *Br J Sports Med*. 2019 [cited 2019 May 17];bjsports-2019–100685. Available from: http://bjsm.bmj.c om/lookup/doi/10.1136/bjsports-2019–100685

17. Reardon CL. Psychiatric comorbidities in sports. *Neurol Clin*. 2017 [cited 2018 Apr 20];35(3):537–46. Available from: www.nc bi.nlm.nih.gov/pubmed/28673414

18. Hainline B, Reardon CL. Breaking a taboo: why the International Olympic Committee convened experts to develop a consensus statement on mental health in elite athletes. *Br J Sports Med*. 2019;bjsports-2019–100681.

19. Glick ID, Stillman MA, Reardon CL, Ritvo EC. Managing psychiatric issues in elite athletes. *J Clin Psychiatry* . 2012 [cited 2016 Dec 7];73(05):640–4. Available from: http://article.psychiatrist.com/? ContentType=START&ID=10007876

20. Kamm R. The sport psychiatry examination. In: Begel D, Burton RW, eds. *Sport Psychiatry*. New York. WW Norton. 2000. p. 159–90.

21. Kamm RL. Interviewing principles for the psychiatrically aware sports medicine physician. *Clin Sports Med* . 2005 [cited 2016 Nov 21];24(4):745–69. Available from: http://linkinghub.elsevier.com/retrie ve/pii/S0278591905000463

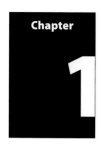

American Football: Cognitive Impairment

Thomas McCabe, Willie Stewart, Mayur Pandya and Joe Kasper

Athlete expert advisor: Steve Sanders

In collision sports there is ongoing ethical and scientific debate on the relevance and significance of previous heavy physical contact burden and, specifically, previous head injuries and the possible neuropsychiatric effects on the ageing athlete.

A sports psychiatrist with expertise in the evaluation of cognitive dysfunction is well placed to assess athletes who present with changes in behaviour and especially when classic short-term memory deficits may not be obvious on initial assessment. Atypical presentations may be found with onset in later life; changes in social function may be specific to the life stage and patient expectations may be different. Treatment options may put greater emphasis on social interventions and pharmacological options differ from those used in a younger individual.

The majority of players retire from elite sport before the age of 40, yet their sporting identity can remain a strong component of their sense of self and contribute to their quality of life for many years. The complexity of interaction between physical and cognitive decline, adjustment to a post-sporting life and social problems experienced in older adults often require collaboration between many professionals and a multidisciplinary approach to treatment and care.

Background

FB is a 53-year-old Caucasian male living in the USA. He had played professional football in the NFL until his thirties and in retirement had worked as a coach. He has two grown-up children who have now left home. He is not currently working and lives with his wife of 28 years. He was initially reviewed by his family doctor in response to his wife's concerns. Although his participation in this initial consultation was minimal it was noted that his personality seemed to have coarsened and there were significant changes in his behaviour. As a result he was referred to a psychiatrist for a more detailed assessment. He only agreed to attend this assessment after much encouragement from his family and friends although he had admitted privately to a friend that 'something was not quite right'. The report from this psychiatric assessment is set out below.

Presenting Complaint

F: 'I'm not sure what all the fuss is about, everything is fine with me.'

WIFE: 'He's a different man from before and is completely unpredictable.'

History of Presenting Complaint

F's wife reported that over the past five years his moods had been very 'up and down'. More recently over the past two years she had felt 'on edge' around him and feared making him angry. She had not considered a medical cause for this, until recently.

His wife provided the majority of this initial history, although FB participated as rapport improved and he responded more openly to questioning as the consultation progressed.

F had retired from professional football 18 years earlier at the age of 35. After struggling with the transition out of professional sport, he began working as a coach for his college team alongside an old team-mate. His players loved his infectious and 'fiery' demeanour and he would regularly let off some steam at his players and match officials. However, his wife noted him to be withdrawn and quiet after training and games, with little meaningful conversation in the evenings. She put this down to him having a busy schedule and tried to get him to socialise more with family and friends, and this seemed to work initially. F held this position for 12 years before voluntarily stepping down. He said he left because he lost his 'passion' to coach. In hindsight, this was when his wife had noticed deterioration in his behaviour.

Since leaving this coaching position, he had not looked for employment again and as he was financially comfortable he had intended to engage more with family life and find other hobbies. His wife reported that he had not 'done much of anything since then'. F often stayed up late watching TV, which he had seldom if ever done previously. It greatly concerned his wife that he now rarely left the family home unless he was with someone. She was concerned at how agitated he could become even in previously familiar surroundings. His wife had hoped he would 'snap out of it'. She admitted to 'putting up with him' and only considered going to the doctor in recent months, as things had got unbearable for her and she described that 'he needs almost constant supervision'.

F's behaviour had also become unpredictable in company over the past six months and he had embarrassed his wife with inappropriate sexualised comments during their infrequent social occasions. He could become irritable at the slightest change to his routine around the home (e.g. food choices, bed time and unexpected visitors). She felt she could calm him down but this was taking longer and longer to achieve. His wife thought this had been a general gradual decline rather than a sudden deterioration.

On 'good days', F enjoyed talking about 'the old times' when friends occasionally visited and he continued to watch and enjoy most sports on TV. He felt able to follow the game plans and was able to comment on tactics. His wife had noticed that he had started to have difficulty finding the sporting channels on the TV.

F said he felt low and rated his mood at 6/10. He still enjoyed some of his usual activities and denied any daytime fatigue or sleep difficulties. He did admit to boredom when at home and would like to get out of his house more but had no specific plans on how to achieve this. When directly asked, he was adamant there were no issues with his memory, concentration or perceptions. He easily recounted his sporting career and remembered scores from specific games from many years previously but struggled to recall recent games he had watched on TV and this caused some embarrassment and agitation.

F said that he thought his family were overreacting although he did not have an explanation for their observations.

His wife was asked directly if she had noticed any repetitive movements, ritualistic or compulsive behaviours or any altered food preferences but denied that any of these features were present.

Past Psychiatric History

He had never previously had any mental health problems. Specifically, he had never had treatment with any psychiatric medication and no periods of psychiatric hospitalisation.

Family History

His maternal grandmother had dementia and towards the end of her life had required intensive nursing care for over two years.

Past Medical History

Hypertension well controlled with medication.

Arthritis in both knees and in the small joints of his hands.

During his professional sporting career he had numerous rib fractures but without long-term complications, corrective surgery on his right achilles tendon, a meniscectomy in right knee, and a right biceps tendon repair.

F reported numerous concussions over his playing career. He admitted that he would often minimise or not report symptoms to avoid being taken out of play. He thought he had experienced approximately '20 or 30' in varying degrees of severity. Residual post-concussive symptoms commonly included headaches, light-sensitivity, nausea and dizziness. Symptoms ranged from 2–15 days in duration. He denied loss of consciousness with any of his concussions. In the final two years of his professional career he had begun experiencing chronic headaches, which dissipated when he retired.

Medication

No known drug allergies

Angiotensin-converting enzyme inhibitor (for hypertension)

Topical anti-inflammatory

His wife sets his medication out for him daily and monitors his adherence

Social History

F has been married to his wife for 28 years and they live in their own home together. She did charity work through her church as a regular hobby but of late had become reluctant to leave her husband alone for any significant period of time. They have two adult children who are both in their twenties and have moved away from the family home.

He drank the occasional glass of red wine with food although was a non-smoker and denied any recreational drug use.

Personal History

F described his childhood experiences as 'simple'. He grew up in a small rural town where his father was a farmer and his mother a part-time waitress. He had one younger sister and continued to have a good relationship with her. He said that he was 'hyper' as a young child and consequently his parents encouraged him into sports, primarily as a means to release some of his excess energy. Academically he was an average student.

His passion for his sport was prioritised over academic studies throughout school. He began playing football at age 10 and in high school played as a running back. At college he was switched to playing defence where he received national attention for his superb speed and aggressive style of play. He played in this role for the rest of his professional career.

Pre-Morbid Personality

He described himself as an extroverted person and enjoyed socialising with peers. His wife agreed with this.

Forensic History

There was no formal contact with the police although 18 months previously he was given a ride home following an isolated drinking session in a local bar with former team-mates.

Collateral History

Before the conclusion of F's evaluation, his wife was interviewed alone. She admitted she 'should have done something about this long before now, I've let him down'. She added that he had displayed more hypersexual tendencies, in the form of frequent demands for sex from her. He had also accused her of being unfaithful.

Four weeks earlier, she had contacted the police after he aggressively confronted her. No further action was taken as the situation was defused with the police presence. This incident was the main catalyst for her decision to pursue a psychiatric assessment.

F's son and daughter visit approximately twice a year. On the most recent visit, they noticed a change in their father's short-term memory. They had expressed concerns with regards to his behaviour previously but he would always dismiss this. His son reported that his father had become repetitive in conversation and had noticed him misplacing several items during his most recent stay. F's wife had not observed any obvious signs of disorientation in memory although on reflection felt he might be covering up any deficits. His daughter had also noticed that he had stopped helping out around the kitchen with meal preparation and other chores as he used to. He had also twice left the shower on without noticing. He had stopped texting his daughter and now preferred to phone her when getting in contact. F was largely dismissive of any memory issues although did appreciate he may have had 'one too many head knocks back in the day'.

Mental State Examination

F presented as taller than average and muscular. He appeared older than his age. He was dressed casually in jeans and a shirt. His hygiene and grooming were reasonable although he had several small shaving cuts on his chin and cheek. No involuntary movements or tremor were observed. His gait was slow and deliberate and he displayed appropriate eye contact although with a rather blank expression at times. He enquired of the assessor's name and qualifications on three occasions and looked to his wife for reassurance throughout the assessment. He mostly laughed off any lapses in short-term memory or pauses to collect his thoughts. His demeanour was generally calm and cooperative during the interview, although there were a few instances of mild irritation and defensiveness when concerns over changes in memory were raised. F was able to follow basic instructions. His speech was of normal tone; however, there was evidence of word-finding difficulty and repetitive content – particularly of his past sporting career. He swore occasionally in a non-aggressive way and would then quickly apologise. His mood was reported as 'great', while his affect appeared dysthymic with limited variability. His thoughts were concrete in nature, focusing on being assessed by a psychiatrist, and periodically required redirection. There was no obvious delusional thought content and he was not obviously responding to any external stimuli. His insight was limited with regards to any possible ongoing mental illness and in particular he downplayed or denied any problems with his memory and mood.

Risk Assessment

Self: He had not expressed any suicidal intent or plan and there was no history of such behaviours. His wife gave him medication, which was locked away in a cupboard as he had become disorganised previously and at risk of either non-adherence or unintentional overdose. There had been no instances of wandering during the night and he was accompanied by his wife throughout the majority of the day and when outside his home, which minimised the risk of any wandering or disorientation. His wife had taken over management of the family finances.

Others: Recent escalation in irritability and verbally aggressive confrontations with his wife. He did not have access to firearms. He had stopped driving his car at the request of his wife.

Protective factors: He recognised that something was 'not quite right' and had agreed to attend in order for this to be assessed and to stop driving. He had a caring and attentive family environment. F was not using any disinhibiting agents e.g. illicit drugs or high consumption of alcohol.

Physical Examination

Pulse and blood pressure were in the normal range (pulse 68 bpm and blood pressure 136/84). Pupils equal and reactive and fundoscopy showed no pathological cupping of the discs. Orientated to person, place, time and situation. Speech was mildly dysarthric but comprehension was intact. Upper extremity exam notable for mild bilateral rigidity, bradykinesia and progressive slowness and amplitude of rapid alternating movements. No intention tremor. No clear asymmetry. Finger-to-nose testing was non-fluid. Unable to maintain balance during pull testing.

Investigations

Laboratory investigations: normal full blood count, thyroid, liver and renal function. Elevated triglycerides and total cholesterol. Infection markers normal (including C-reactive protein).

Urine dipstick was clear with no protein or glucose.

Neurocognitive testing: Montreal Cognitive Assessment (MoCA) 19/30

Visuospatial 3/5

Naming 1/3

Attention 4/6

Language 3/3

Abstraction 0/2

Memory 2/5

Orientation 6/6

(The MoCA is a scoring tool used to assist clinicians with patients who may have a dementia illness. It tests a variety of cognitive domains as set out above. 'Normal controls' would be expect to score between 27 and 30 points and a score below 18 would be considered evidence of an ongoing dementia syndrome.)

Neurocognitive testing: Frontal Assessment Battery (FAB)

Similarities – 2

Lexical fluency – 2

Luria Test – 2

Conflicting instructions – 1

Go No Go Test – 2

Prehension Behaviour – 1

(The FAB is a tool that can be used at the bedside or in a clinic setting to assist in discriminating between dementias with a frontal lobe predominance and dementia of Alzheimer's type. The FAB has validity in distinguishing fronto-temporal-type dementia from Alzheimer's dementia in mildly impaired patients (Mini Mental State Examination (MMSE) > 24). Total score is from a maximum of 18, higher scores indicating better performance.)

Neuroimaging: MRI brain imaging performed one month previously showed generalised cortical atrophy, with mild hippocampal volume loss.

Case Formulation

F presented as a 53-year-old Caucasian male and a former professional NFL player. There had been an insidious onset of unpredictable behaviour and decline in cognitive function that had become more apparent since retirement from coaching. The symptoms of unpredictability and aggression had led to acute safety concerns expressed by family members and led them to pursue a clinical opinion on his change in behaviour. A decline in activities of daily living was noted from the collateral history. Reliance on others had contributed to F becoming frustrated at his ability to attend to his own needs. He appeared to be largely apathetic to any ongoing concerns expressed by others.

A family history of dementia (second degree relative) suggested a possible genetic component to his condition. His previous occupation had exposed him to repeated head traumas which may not have been recognised, disclosed or been partially evaluated at the time. He did not appear to have an educational background that would minimise any cognitive deficits ('cognitive reserve').

Deficits on formal cognitive assessment were noted with frontal lobe predominance. The combined history, objective cognitive testing and basic neuroimaging would suggest F had an unspecified dementia syndrome. On account of his age, this could be as a result of early-onset Alzheimer's dementia, vascular dementia or the behavioural variant fronto-temporal dementia. Chronic traumatic encephalopathy (CTE) and traumatic brain injury (TBI) would also form part of the differential diagnosis. He had presented relatively late negating the possibility of early interventions.

Plan

- A safety plan was discussed and agreed with the patient and his family, who were also given information on his possible diagnosis. F's wife was given information on how to optimise living conditions at home to reduce the potential for falls and minimise the risk of wandering, and was given orientation aids for around the home. F's wife discussed possible triggers for increased agitation and a plan for help, should this be unmanageable, was agreed
- F was referred to an occupational therapist for a functional assessment to assist with domestic needs
- He reluctantly agreed to a further referral to a neurologist for consideration of additional investigations such as Single-Photon Emission Computed Tomography scan (SPECT) and lumbar puncture (for tau and amyloid-beta). This referral would assist with diagnostic dementia subtyping and attempt to rule out any rarer organic cause for the presentation, such as variant Creutzfeldt-Jakob disease or Lewy body dementia
- An outpatient follow-up review with the assessing psychiatrist was arranged for one month's time

Questions

Q 1   Which statements are correct regarding CTE?
   A. Cavum septum pellucidum is a common finding
   B. Neurofibrillary tangles typically cluster in the depths of cortical sulci
   C. CTE has only been described in individuals exposed to repetitive brain injury
   D. CTE is synonymous with dementia pugilistica and symptoms may include emotional lability, memory impairment and ataxia
   E. Although tau pathologies are typical of CTE, other neuropathology patterns may co-exist

Q 2   Which of the following investigations will allow a definitive diagnosis of CTE to be made in this case?
   A. Cerebrospinal fluid phospho-tau and amyloid-beta assessment
   B. Positron emission tomography (PET) studies for tau
   C. Functional MRI
   D. Post-mortem examination of the brain
   E. The proposed SPECT studies

Q 3   CTE is associated with exposure to repetitive mild traumatic brain injury/concussion. Of the following, which is known to be associated with lower concussion risk within sport?
A. Protective headgear, such as football helmets
B. Age under 18
C. History of previous concussion
D. Artificial football pitches
E. Male versus female sex

Q 4   Answer true or false to the following statements:
A. A majority of former NFL players will develop CTE
B. There is no effective therapy for CTE
C. Historically, suicide rates are known to be higher than anticipated in former NFL players
D. CTE was first described in 2005
E. Cases of CTE have been described in individuals with no known exposure to brain injury or contact sports

Q 5   Choose the correct statements regarding management of neuropsychiatric symptoms (NPS) and persistent concussive symptoms:
A. All forms of psychiatric medications are absolutely contraindicated in those experiencing NPS in concussion
B. There are low levels of empirical data to guide psychiatric treatment after single or repetitive concussions
C. A biopsychosocial formulation and management plan for NPS should be followed for athletes with persistent concussive symptoms and NPS
D. Medication should only be prescribed if licensed for NPS in persistent concussion symptoms
E. Graded, sub-maximal aerobic exercise may help athletes towards post-concussive recovery

Answers

Q 1) A, B, D, E

Clinical observations of the chronic neuropsychiatric outcomes of former boxers in the early part of the twentieth century led to the first descriptions of what was then referred to as the 'punch-drunk' syndrome (1). In the decades that followed, a typical syndrome of psychiatric symptoms, emotional lability, personality changes, memory impairment and dementia, pyramidal and extrapyramidal dysfunction and cerebellar impairment was described (2). Neuropathological studies over the latter half of that century defined and named the pathology as dementia pugilistica (3, 4).

With more recent recognition of this pathology in a range of athletes in sports other than boxing (5–10), and in those surviving exposure to a single moderate or severe traumatic brain injury (11,12), the term 'chronic traumatic encephalopathy' (CTE) has replaced 'dementia pugilistica'. Neuropathological consensus criteria for the assessment and diagnosis of the pathology associated with CTE have been defined (13). These describe common abnormalities in the septum pellucidum, either as cavum or fenestrated septum, together with histological evidence of CTE neuropathologic change (CTE-NC) in a typical pattern and distribution of hyperphosphorylated tau (p-tau) pathology. P-tau pathologies in CTE-NC typically appear as patchy cortical deposits in neurons and glia. In early series on the pathology of boxers, neurofibrillary tangles containing p-tau were described with a distribution to the medial temporal lobe (4). Later series noted a more patchy distribution of pathology, often clustered at the depths of cortical sulci, and with apparent preferential involvement of superficial cortical layers.

Despite a majority of case series describing pathology in symptomatic former athletes, CTE-NC can be encountered in apparently cognitively intact 'normal' controls. A review of tissue samples from the Queen Square Brain Bank (London, UK) identified CTE-NC in 12% of cases whether or not there was a history of neurodegenerative disease (14).

While tau pathologies are typical of CTE-NC, multiple other pathologies have also been found in material from former contact/collision sport athletes and a number of other neuro-degeneration associated proteinopathies are recognised in CTE. Amyloid-beta (A-beta) pathologies are commonly described alongside p-tau pathologies from the earliest descriptions in boxers (15) to more recent case series in non-boxer athletes (10, 11,16). Notably, the prevalence of A-beta plaque pathology in CTE increases with increasing age at death and is more commonly encountered where there are clinical symptoms of cognitive impairment (16).

The emerging picture is of a complex pathology in which CTE-NC may be the primary dementia-associated pathology, often with multiple other co-morbid pathologies present. CTE-NC may also be a co-morbid pathology in the context of an alternative dementia diagnosis or may represent as an incidental pathology in an otherwise asymptomatic patient (10).

Q 2) D

Although preliminary consensus criteria for the neuropathological assessment and diagnosis of CTE-NC are agreed (13), no such consensus criteria for the clinical diagnosis of CTE have been defined. As such, definitive diagnosis of CTE requires post-mortem examination with formal neuropathological assessment. In this context, imaging studies remain of limited value; their role being in assisting in the elimination of potentially treatable alternative diagnoses and in narrowing differential diagnosis in suspected neurodegenerative disease. In patients with possible CTE, structural imaging may show abnormalities in the septum pellucidum (17) and atrophy of the medial temporal lobe, but neither is pathognomonic for the condition.

Although the pattern and distribution of p-tau pathologies in CTE-NC are regarded as sufficiently distinct to be pathognomonic of the disease, to date, PET imaging studies have not succeeded in exploiting this pathology for secure in vivo diagnostic purposes. Nevertheless, various radiolabelled tau ligands are under review, and although preliminary data from limited case series hold some promise none have reached clinical practice.

While fluid biomarkers have been extensively researched in wider neurodegenerative disease, in particular Alzheimer's disease (AD) (18), there is considerably less experience in CTE. In patients with AD, high levels of total- and phosphorylated-tau and low levels of

A-beta42 are documented in early phases and at diagnosis. However, thus far, only limited studies in small numbers of former athletes have been pursued, with no clear indication of utility in CTE diagnosis (19).

Q 3) E

Studies exploring the utility of various forms of protective equipment, including headgear, across a range of sports have failed to demonstrate any robust data to suggest any benefit in reducing concussion risk. Many are confounded by poor study design, inconsistent definition of injury and low subject numbers (20). However, helmets do provide benefit in reducing risk of focal head injuries (21, 22), and remain recommended in activities such as ice hockey, ski-ing and cycling.

Regarding other risk-modifying factors in concussion, data confirm that younger age and history of previous concussion are associated with increased injury risk (23). Further, younger individuals are at particular risk of catastrophic outcome from apparently mild TBI/concussion through a rare complication known as diffuse brain swelling, sometimes referred to colloquially as 'second impact syndrome' (24). The pathophysiology of this condition remains uncertain. It appears to be a particular risk in adolescents and hence concussion management in younger age groups is typically more conservative.

Female athletes are recognised as being at increased risk of concussion when compared to male athletes (23); an observation that is supported by data across several sports where participation rules are equivalent for male and female players. The reasons for this are uncertain, although may include the recognised structural differences between male and female axons perhaps resulting in axons in females being more at risk of injury under dynamic loading (25).

Q 4) F/T/F/F/T

Although coming to wider attention with the first description of CTE-NC in a former American footballer in 2005 (5), neither the pathology nor the term CTE originate in this century. First descriptions of the neuropathology of former boxers date to the middle of the last century (26). To date, there are fewer than 400 confirmed cases of CTE-NC in the literature (27). Current reporting in CTE is based on descriptions of brains examined after death as the diagnosis can only be made at post-mortem examination. Inherent biases in case donations and the limitations of small samples mean that no meaningful data on disease prevalence can be obtained. Nevertheless, interpretations of limited studies reporting high prevalence of CTE-NC in their series (28) have led to a belief that CTE is common among certain former athlete cohorts.

Despite first formal description of the 'punch-drunk' syndrome in 1928 (1), studies to identify rates of neurodegenerative disease in former athletes suffer from multiple limitations, including study design and small numbers. Regarding American Football, while a threefold increase in neurodegenerative mortality has been described for a cohort of former NFL players (29), studies in former high school footballers fail to identify increased dementia risk (30). There remains no robust data to allow interpretation of CTE prevalence in populations at risk, let alone sufficient data to suggest that a majority of athletes might develop the disease.

In contrast to early accounts of CTE in former boxers, more contemporary reports of non-boxer athletes describe suicidality, aggression and disinhibition among psychiatric symptomatology. Indeed, there is a perception that former contact sports athletes exposed to repetitive mild traumatic brain injury are at increased risk of suicide. However, this appears to be based on multiple high-profile media reports rather than on unbiased scientific studies. Although recent studies might suggest a higher than anticipated suicide rate among individuals with autopsy identified CTE-NC (28), this is not supported by population data, and in a study of retired American NFL players the suicide rate was lower than in an equivalent general population sample (31).

While no effective therapy for CTE is recognised, neither is there a robust strategy for its diagnosis. Therapies directed at managing potentially treatable conditions remain the mainstay for individuals thought to be at high risk of CTE and this includes treatment of pre-existing or co-morbid mental health disorders.

Q 5)   B, C and E

Despite the high frequency of concussion within sport, there is limited empirical data on psychiatric treatment following single or repeated TBI (32). Like other areas of sports psychiatry where evidence is extrapolated from the general population, NPS care should follow these same treatment principles.

Examples of biological factors that need to be explored include the presence of medical, psychiatric and substance misuse co-morbidity. Clinicians should review for any tolerability or compliance issues related to previous psychotropic or analgesic medications. Also, any history of previous concussive episodes and associated dizziness may indicate a higher risk of re-injury susceptibility and delayed recovery (33). Some studies have suggested that genetic polymorphisms related to plasticity and repair (APOE), calcium influx (CACNA1E), synaptic connectivity (GRIN2A), and uptake and deposit of glutamate (SLC17A7) may act as biomarkers for concussion incidence and recovery (33). Psychosocial and cultural factors that should be considered include the patient's current relationships, stressors and social support.

Until recently, athletes suffering from concussion were generally advised to rest completely in the period following injury until symptomology resolved. Guidance and practice have changed in recent years, with emerging evidence suggesting aerobic exercise as a non-pharmacological treatment for patients with post-concussive symptoms (34). Return of baseline exercise tolerance through graded exercise rehabilitation (adapted from the Buffalo Concussion Treadmill Test) may provide a physiological biomarker towards post-concussive recovery (35).

Most psychiatric medications for persistent concussive NPS symptoms will be prescribed 'off-label'. In keeping with general prescribing principles, prescribers should 'start low, go slow, but go' to reduce brain sensitivity issues following brain injury. Also, medication combinations that lower seizure threshold, cause weight gain, create dependence and require excessive 'as required' administration should be avoided.

There is a paucity of well-designed, comparative trials to guide psychiatric medication prescription in NPS and concussion (36). Table 1.1 outlines NPS treatment options based on current clinical consensus.

Table 1.1 Psychiatric medication options for NPS post-concussion (adapted from Rao V et al. 2017)

Psychotropic Medication	Example	Target Symptoms
Antidepressants	Selective serotonin reuptake inhibitors (SSRIs) e.g. sertraline 25–150mg Serotonin noradrenergic reuptake inhibitors (SNRI) Venlafaxine ER 37.5–225mg Duloxetine 30-90mg	Depression Anxiety Aggression, agitation
Mood Stabilisers	Sodium valproate 125mg–1g Carbamazepine 100–600mg	Mood cycling
Atypical Antipsychotics	Quetiapine 25–200mg Risperidone 0.5–4mg	Psychosis Aggression, agitation Mood cycling Irritability
Dopamine Agonists	Methylphenidate 5–20mg	Inattention, mental fatigue
Acetylcholinesterase Inhibitors	Donepezil 5–10mg	Memory loss
Anxiolytics	Buspirone 10–60mg	Anxiety Irritability
Beta Blockers	Propanolol 30–120mg	Aggression

Summary of the Chapter and the Topics Covered

- Issues related to retirement following professional sport
- Assessment and management of cognitive impairment related to repeated head injuries
- Clinical tools used to assess cognitive impairment
- Risk assessment and biopsychosocial management options for cognitive impairment
- Challenges related to CTE diagnosis
- Pharmacological options for NPS post-concussion

References

1. Martland H. Punch drunk. *J Am Med Assoc.* (1928);91:1103–07.

2. Roberts G. *Brain Damage in Boxers: A Study of the Prevalence of Traumatic Encephalopathy Among Ex-Professional Boxers.* London: Pitman; 1969.

3. Corsellis JA Bruton CJ Freeman-Browne D. The aftermath of boxing. *Psychol Med.* (1973);3;270–303.

4. Smith, DH, Johnson, VE, Stewart, W. Chronic neuropathologies of single and repetitive TBI: Substrates of dementia? *Nat Rev Neurol.* 2013;9:211–21.

5. Omalu BI, et al. Chronic traumatic encephalopathy in a National Football League player. *Neurosurgery.* 2005;57:128–33.

6. McKee AC, Cantu RC, Nowinski CJ, et al. Chronic traumatic encephalopathy in athletes: Progressive tauopathy after

repetitive head injury. *J Neuropathol Exp Neurol.* 2009;68:709–35.

7. Stewart W, McNamara PH, Lawlor B, Hutchinson S, Farrell M. Chronic traumatic encephalopathy: A potential late and under recognized consequence of rugby union. *QJM.* 2016;109:11–15.

8. Hay J, Johnson VE, Smith DH, Stewart W. Chronic traumatic encephalopathy: The neuropathological legacy of traumatic brain injury. *Ann Rev Pathol.* 2016;11:21–45.

9. Ling H. et al. Mixed pathologies including chronic traumatic encephalopathy account for dementia in retired association football (soccer) players. *Acta Neuropathol.* 2017;133: 337–52.

10. Lee, EB, Kinch, K, Johnson, VE, Trojanowski, JQ, Smith, DH, Stewart, W. Chronic traumatic encephalopathy is a common co-morbidity, but less frequent primary dementia in former soccer and rugby players. *Acta Neuropathol.* 2019. doi.org/10.1007/s00401-019-02030-y

11. Johnson VE, Stewart JE, Stewart W, Smith, DH. Widespread tau and amyloid-beta pathology many years after a single traumatic brain injury in humans. *Brain Pathol.* 2012;22:142–9.

12. Zanier ER, Bertani I, Sammali E, et al. Induction of a transmissible tau pathology by traumatic brain injury. *Brain.* 2018;141:2685–99.

13. McKee, A, Cairns, NJ, Dickson, et al. The first NINDS/NIBIB consensus meeting to define neuropathological criteria for the diagnosis of chronic traumatic encephalopathy. *Acta Neuropathol.* 2016;131:75–86.

14. Ling, H, Holton,JL, Shaw,K, et al. Histological evidence of chronic traumatic encephalopathy in a large series of neurodegenerative diseases. *Acta Neuropathol.* 2015;130:891–3.

15. Roberts, GW, Allsop, D, Bruton, C. The occult aftermath of boxing. *J Neurol Neurosurg Psychiatry.* 1990; 53:373–8.

16. Stein, TD, Montenigro, PH, Alvarez, VE, Xia, W, Crary, JF, Tripodis, Y, et al. Beta-amyloid deposition in chronic traumatic encephalopathy. *Acta Neuropathol.* 2015;130:1–34.

17. Koerte, IK, Hufschmidt, J, Muehlmann, M, et al. Cavum Septi Pellucidi in symptomatic former professional football players. *J Neurotrauma.* 2016;33:346–53.

18. Blennow, K. A review of fluid biomarkers for Alzheimer's disease: Moving from CSF to blood. *Neurol Ther.* 2017;6:S15-S24.

19. Alosco, ML, Tripodis, Y, Fritts, NG et al. Cerebrospinal fluid tau, Aβ, and sTREM2 in former National Football League players: Modeling the relationship between repetitive head impacts, microglial activation, and neurodegeneration. *Alzheimers Dement.* 2018;14:1159–70.

20. Emery, CA, Black, AM, Kolstad, A, et al. What strategies can be used to effectively reduce the risk of concussion in sport? A systematic review. *Br J Sports Med.* 2016;51:978–84.

21. Marshall SW, Waller AE, Dick RW, et al. An ecologic study of protective equipment and injury in two contact sports. *Int J Epidemiol.* 2002;31:587–92.

22. Hagel BE, Pless IB, Goulet C, et al. Effectiveness of helmets in skiers and snowboarders: Case-control and case crossover study. *BMJ.* 2005;330:281.

23. McCrory, P, Meeuwisse, WH, Aubry, A et al. Consensus statement on concussion in sport: The 4th International Conference on Concussion in Sport held in Zurich November 2012. *Br J Sports Med.* 2012;47:250–8.

24. Saunders RL, Harbaugh RE. The second impact in catastrophic contact-sports head trauma. *JAMA.* 1984;252:538–9.

25. Dolle, JP, Jave, A, Anderson, SA, Ahmadzadeh, H, Shenov, VB, Smith, DH. Newfound sex differences in axonal structure underlie differential outcomes from in vitro traumatic axonal injury. *Exp Neurol.* 2018;300:121–34.

26. Brandenburg W, Hallervorden J. Dementia pugilistica with anatomical findings. *Virchows Archiv.* 1954; 325:680–709.

27. Smith, DH, Johnson, VE, Trojanowski, JQ, Stewart, W. Chronic traumatic encephalopathy: Confusion and controversies. *Nat Rev Neurol.* 2019;15:179–83.

28. Mez, J, Daneshvar, DH, Kiernan, PT, Abdolmohammadi, B, Alvarez, VE, Huber, BR et al. Clinicopathological evaluation of chronic traumatic encephalopathy in players of American football. *JAMA.* 2017;318:360–70.

29. Lehman, EJ, Hein, MJ, Baron, SL and Gersic, CM. Neurodegenerative causes of death among retired National Football League players. *Neurology.* 2012;79:1970–4.

30. Janssen, PHH, et al. High school football and late-life risk of neurodegenerative syndromes, 1956–1970. *Mayo Clin. Proc.* 2017;92:66–71.

31. Lehman, EJ, Hein, MJ, Gersic, CM. Suicide mortality among retired National Football League players who played 5 or more seasons. *An J Sports Med.* 2016;44:2486–91.

32. Rao V, et al. Neuropsychiatric aspects of concussion: Acute and chronic sequelae. *Concussion* 2017;2(1):CNC29.

33. McDevitt J and Krynetskiy E. Genetic findings in sport-related concussions: Potential for individualized medicine? *Concussion.* 2017; 2(1). https://doi.org/10.2217/cnc-2016-0020

34. Leddy JJ, Haider MN, Ellis M, Willer BS. Exercise is medicine for concussion. *Curr Sports Med Rep.* 2018;17(8):262–70.

35. Leddy JJ, Kozlowski K, Fung M, Pendergast DR, Willer B. Regulatory and autoregulatory physiological dysfunction as a primary characteristic of post concussion syndrome: Implications for treatment. *Neurorehabilitation.* 2007;22(3):199–205.

36. Warden DL, Gordon B, McAllister TW et al. Guidelines for the pharmacological treatment of neurobehavioural episodes of traumatic brain injury. *J Neurotrauma.* 2006;23(10):1468–501.

Athletics: Energy Levels, Exercise Addiction and Disordered Eating

Emily Dudgeon, Renee McGregor and Rebecca Robinson

Psychiatric assessments of endurance athletes commonly identify symptoms of anxiety, compulsive behaviours, overtraining and eating disorders. There is often overlap in how these issues present and there can be diagnostic challenges. Concurrent physical injury and delayed presentation to mental health services can further complicate the presenting picture. The sports psychiatrist needs to be aware of why endurance athletes are at risk of overtraining and under-fuelling, should be able to identify the associated psychiatric and medical conditions and would expect to work as part of a multidisciplinary team in supporting the athlete towards recovery. Increased awareness among athletes themselves, their family, friends and coaching teams can help to prevent the athlete becoming energy deficient and can reduce the likelihood of emotional difficulties progressing to more serious problems or even mental illness.

Background

BR presented as a 22-year-old single, university student and an endurance runner. She had competed successfully at middle- and long-distance events since the age of 14. Since transitioning to university, B had increased her training load considerably with the hope of competing at national level and eventual selection for international competition. However, over the past year she had suffered two stress fractures that had not been given appropriate time to heal. Initially, she had presented to her primary healthcare physician (GP) several times including for ongoing pain management, which she was attempting to treat herself by way of over-the-counter medications. During one of these GP consultations, she revealed how stressed and anxious she was and the effect this had on her athletic performance. She was then referred to a sports psychiatrist, based on the perceived longevity of untreated mental health symptoms and her wish to return to competitive sport as soon as possible. The report from this consultation and assessment is below.

Presenting Complaint

'I can't handle not being able to run, I feel so low and anxious.'

History of Presenting Complaint

B started out as a cross-country runner and progressed to track athletics. She first competed at the English Schools Championships when she was 15 and felt that she could aim to compete for her country as a junior (under-20) athlete. When she went to university she joined a successful training group and significantly increased the volume and intensity of training. She quickly made big improvements in her personal best times across a range of distances. However she started to experience a 'niggling' pain in her right foot. She trained through this for a few weeks without telling anyone until her coach noticed her limping and suggested she consult a doctor. An x-ray suggested a navicular stress fracture and this was confirmed by MRI. Conservative management was recommended after an orthopaedic consultation. She reluctantly agreed to this approach but on reflection wished she had taken a surgical option that would have meant less time away from running.

During her enforced rest she had begun investigating how to manage her weight, as she feared gaining weight and any detrimental effect this might have on her performance. She had always been quite regimented with her meals although she ate a varied diet. She decided to avoid meals if she was not hungry and to completely cut out anything that she thought was high in fat. She began to weigh herself regularly every week to monitor for any increase.

She cross-trained hard to maintain her fitness with the motivation of being able to come back over the summer when her injury had improved. However, when she began running again she developed shin pain. She initially thought this was simply 'shin splints' but the pain eventually became unbearable even after just a few minutes of running. She was prompted by her coach to see her doctor and an x-ray revealed a new stress fracture, this time in her tibia. B went back to see the same orthopaedic doctor and was advised to take an extended break from training and then a graduated return to running after three months. She thought that the second injury was simply bad luck and that her doctors did not understand her desire to run and her ambitions. After a period of rest lasting two to three weeks she began cross-training intensely with the intention of making up for her lack of a GB junior (under-20) vest by gaining selection for the under-23 team. Her coach was unaware of these extra and unsupervised training sessions. In addition, she was monitoring her diet even more closely and missing occasional meals if she felt she was likely to gain weight or looked 'too fat' when she saw herself in the mirror at the gym. She was now lighter than when she came to university with a weight of 50kg and body mass index (BMI) of 17.7 but often thought she would be even faster if she were lighter still.

She finished second in the national championships and gained international selection for the under-23 team. She believed this validated her view that she knew more about how to train her own body than others including her coach and her doctor. However, shortly after this her progress slowed. She was struggling to motivate herself for the first time and was increasingly picking up minor illnesses. She suspected she might be anaemic or have another underlying illness that was stopping her training from bringing about the improvements she expected. B decided to go to the GP for some tests and agreed to stop doing extra training sessions while awaiting the results.

B began to feel generally more anxious both during training and her life outside of running. She felt the need to 'escape' when in company and found herself making excuses to end conversations prematurely. She could not get 'in the zone' anymore when running and had stopped on three occasions after 10 minutes or so in despair, crying and feeling overwhelmed. She described broken sleep, fatigue with frequent evening naps and loss of interest in her studies over the preceding month. She frequently ruminated on whether she would ever get back to her previous levels of performance.

Past Psychiatric History

There was no previous history of any mental health concerns.

Family History

No family history of any mental health problems.

Past Medical History

Amenorrhea – secondary, has not menstruated in previous 10 months, never previously investigated, felt this was a "normal" part of being an athlete.

Right posterior tibial fracture.

Right navicular fracture.

Medication History

Her GP recently suggested using the oral contraceptive pill (OCP) to try to stimulate a hormonal cycle.

Paracetamol 1g, four times daily

Ibuprofen 400mg, three times daily.

Social History

B grew up in a family with one younger and one older sister. Her father is a corporate lawyer and her mother is an accountant. She had made good friends at university but sometimes felt that they did not understand her drive and determination in her sport. She would often get frustrated when they tried to 'distract' her by asking her to go out for a drink, eat unhealthy food or stay up late.

Personal History

B had an unremarkable prenatal period, birth and developmental history. She excelled at school and the head teacher asked her parents to consider moving her up a year but they decided against this. She recalled being popular and enjoyed her time in secondary school. She described it as a busy time during which she was always on her way to another sporting commitment. She got straight As in her exams and fulfilled her desire to go to university to study engineering. B had moved away from home for university. She had never been in a relationship as there was not time and felt this would be a distraction from her academic and sporting aspirations. She got on well with her family but noted that her relationships had become tense because 'my mum doesn't understand what it takes to be an athlete, and is always asking me to train less and eat more'.

Pre-Morbid Personality

She mentioned that she had always been a determined and well-organised person and through this had been successful both academically and in sport. She had often noticed that after a run or other form of exercise she felt happier and less stressed. Recently this feeling had lasted for shorter and shorter periods and sometimes she no longer felt her usual self at all.

Forensic History
There was no history of any offending behaviour.

Collateral History
B declined to allow the psychiatrist to contact her coach or her parents.

Mental State Examination
B was well-kempt but dressed in several jumpers, as if for colder weather than it was. She seemed anxious and restless throughout the consultation. She maintained good eye contact most of the time but appeared withdrawn when asked questions about perceived anxiety. Her speech was normal in rate although low in volume and especially when talking about her anxieties. B reported low mood that was most noticeable when she was not able to carry out her 'normal' training regime. Objectively she appeared euthymic at first but more withdrawn when discussing how she felt when not exercising. There was no delusional thought content but she reported hearing a self-loathing voice that she described as her own thoughts. She reported difficulty concentrating on her studies. She believed there must be an underlying physical illness causing this. She was quite defensive when the intensity of her training was brought up and minimised her injuries and amenorrhea by saying these were not unexpected and that people just do not understand athletes. She saw no link between the intensity of her training and her injuries and general state of health. She dismissed the risks associated with amenorrhea saying 'no serious athlete has a regular menstrual cycle' and 'there is plenty of time to correct that when I have achieved my goals'.

Risk Assessment
Self: She reported having experienced fleeting suicidal ideation but denied any plans or intent. The ideas went away when she exercised and were at their most intense when there had been more than 24 hours without exercise. There was a high risk of further harm through ongoing intense exercise and likely inadequate nutritional intake, particularly as she minimised these harms and did not recognise a link between training, diet and previous harm. There was no risk of harm through substance use and no purging behaviours were described.

Others: No risk of harm to others was reported.

Investigations
- Blood tests carried out by GP (see results below in Table 2.1):
  - Urea and electrolytes
  - Hormonal profile: B hCG, karyotype, thyroid function tests (TFTs), prolactin, follicle stimulating hormone (FSH), luteinizing hormone (LH), oestradiol (E2),

testosterone, sex-hormone binding globulin (SHBG), dehydroepiandrosteron (DHEA), 9am cortisol.
  - Vitamin D
  - Blood glucose, Hba1 c
  - Full blood count
  - Haematinics
  - Liver function tests
  - Gastro screen – coeliac (tTG-IgA), faecal calprotectin (for inflammatory bowel disease)
- Pelvic USS: normal
- DEXA scan: Z score of −1.5

Case Formulation

B is a 22-year-old endurance athlete who has previously competed at a national level since her mid-teens. She presented for the first time with likely relative energy deficiency in sport (RED-S) as well as features of overtraining syndrome (OTS), anxiety, low mood and compulsive exercise. Her energy deficiency may be the result of an eating disorder or disordered eating.

As B's performance level improved, she became particularly focused on running and felt others were not as invested in her career as she was. Importantly, she lacked full insight into the links between her training behaviour, past injuries, anxiety and endocrine dysfunction. B had a significant change in her life circumstances (leaving home and moving from school to university) prior to her injury and did not have the same level of support from her parents as previously. B was high-achieving academically and, along with her successful running career to date, presented as a highly driven and motivated individual who was fearful of losing this. She had been unable to train and compete due to lower leg fractures and this had led to further isolation from her usual support structure.

Plan

- She was reluctant but eventually persuaded of the value of involving her coach in her assessment and care. She was persuaded by the argument that her health and performance were closely linked and that both medical and coaching input would be needed for recovery. She was also reassured that only essential information would be shared and only with her informed consent
- B was referred to a sports nutritionist who was also a qualified dietitian who had worked with athletes with RED-S. The aim was to devise an agreed nutritional plan that would restore and then maintain her energy balance. The frequency of monitoring of her weight was also agreed at this first session
- She was referred to a counsellor with the university health service (supervised by a clinical psychologist) to help her develop a more effective range of emotional regulation techniques and reduce her reliance on exercise as a means of managing her anxiety and low mood. The clinical psychologist would monitor progress and if there were signs of relapse (including the re-emergence of RED-S) a more intensive psychological therapy would be offered (cognitive behavioural therapy for eating disorders)

- She agreed to meet with her coach, a sports medicine doctor who did sessions at the university and her psychiatrist to plan an appropriate volume and intensity of exercise taking into account her health status, energy balance and progress in therapy. These sessions would be repeated every three months during her recovery
- Her blood tests were to be repeated at three months (or sooner if signs of relapse) and her DEXA scan after one year

Questions

Q 1 Examine B's blood results from the hormone profile.

Table 2.1 Blood results

B HCG	Negative
Karyotype	XX
TFTs	TSH low, thyroxine low
Prolactin	High
FSH	Low
LH	Low
E2	Low
Testosterone	Low
SHBG	High
DHEA	Low
Cortisol 9am	High

Which condition are they most representative of?
A. Polycystic Ovarian Syndrome (PCOS)
B. Early menopause
C. RED-S
D. Normal blood results
E. Osteoporosis

Q 2 Which of the below would you consider as part of your management plan for this patient?
A. Hormone replacement therapy
B. Graded return to exercise
C. Psychological support
D. Dietetic support
E. All of the above

Q 3 B lacks insight into her condition and has low mood, mild intermittent suicidal ideation and features of anxiety. What would be the most appropriate way to manage

her psychiatric symptoms with the end goal of restoring her physiological hormonal axes?
A. Anxiolytic pharmacological therapy
B. Cognitive behavioural therapy (CBT)
C. Family therapy
D. Referral to mental health crisis team
E. Advise her on self-management techniques for anxiety e.g. mindfulness

Q 4 Some of the features of addiction may be found in otherwise healthy high-performing athletes. These might include which of the following?
A. Withdrawal phenomena when not exercising
B. Continuing to exercise despite harm
C. Large proportion of time spent exercising
D. Reduction in other activities
E. Tolerance to the effects of exercise

Q 5 B can be fully cleared for return to play (RTP). True or False?

Answers

Q 1) C

Relative energy deficiency in sport (RED-S) is a condition of low energy availability that can impact performance and have long-term adverse consequences on an athlete's physical and mental health. If it occurs during adolescence before bone growth is complete, it can also have a serious impact on growth and development (1). RED-S may develop inadvertently by a simple miscalculation of energy requirements when training is increased or dietary changes are made or it may result from disordered eating or even an eating disorder. B has been restricting her diet to lose weight and has a fear of gaining weight and its consequences. She may also misjudge her shape and appearance and see herself as fat when she is lean. These are the three central features of anorexia nervosa (2). There is no purging and so she would be described as having the restricting subtype and with a BMI > 17 her illness would be in the 'mild' category.

Athletes may present to medical services with amenorrhea, which is classified as primary or secondary. Primary amenorrhea is when menstruation has not started by the age of 16 and secondary amenorrhea is when menstruation ceases after having previously had a regular menstrual cycle. It is important to note that RED-S is just one cause of amenorrhea and other conditions need to be excluded including viral illness such as Epstein-Barr virus, gynaecological conditions, gastrointestinal causes of malabsorption and endocrine conditions such as thyroid disease. Distinguishing RED-S from endocrine disorders can be particularly challenging because of its wide-ranging effects on several of the body's hormonal axes (endocrine axes are inhibited in an effort to conserve energy). Athletes with RED-S may be incorrectly diagnosed with conditions like PCOS without input from a gynaecologist and endocrinologist. PCOS is distinct from RED-S in its hormone profile. PCOS will characteristically cause high testosterone and normal levels of other hormones whereas RED-S causes low testosterone, low LH, low FSH and low E2.

The context provided by history, clinical examination and pelvic ultrasound is essential when considering the cause of amenorrhea. Karyotyping is carried out to rule out conditions such as Turner's syndrome (45, X) and patients who may have gonadal dysgenesis (for example 46, XY karyotype where physical male sexual characteristics do not develop because of androgen insensitivity).

Hormone health is intrinsically linked to energy availability. It has been known since the late 1980s that body weight and percentage of body fat are both contributing factors to whether a woman will start menstruating (adipose tissue plays a vital role in converting androgens to oestrogens) (3). It is now thought that 45 kcal/kg of lean body mass is required to maintain regular menstruation (4). Low body mass and insufficient energy intake also disturb the hypothalamic-gonadal axis in men resulting in a similar syndrome of sporting underperformance, fatigue and loss of libido.

Q 2) E

Given it is defined by low energy availability, the primary treatment of RED-S is to achieve and maintain energy balance. This is likely to involve modifying both eating and training behaviour (5). A proportion of RED-S sufferers are affected by disordered eating and eating disorders, and for these athletes the underlying condition needs to be addressed. This is likely to require more intensive and multidisciplinary support that may include a sports medicine doctor, dietitian, mental health specialist (psychiatrist or clinical psychologist) and the coaching team.

Bone health is intricately linked with sex hormone production, with oestrogen playing a key role in bone homeostasis. Many healthcare professionals prescribe the OCP to amenorrhoeic athletes in an effort to assist with their hormonal dysfunction. However, the OCP masks menstrual disturbance, inhibits ovulation and does not provide adequate bone protection (6). Temporary treatment with hormone replacement therapy while the energy deficit is addressed has been shown to benefit bone health. Particular attention needs to be paid to vitamin D and calcium levels/supplementation given the risk of poor bone health in RED-S sufferers, albeit with an awareness that efficient absorption depends on the presence of oestrogen and testosterone.

Low energy availability may occur due to intentional or unintentional under-fuelling or increased levels of physical activity and either may lead to an energy deficit. Intentional under-fuelling may begin with an athlete paying closer attention to their nutrition that later develops into disordered eating and eventually the full syndrome of an eating disorder. It is well known that athletes have a higher risk than non-athletes of developing eating disorders (7). Initially, athletes may see an improvement in their performance. However, over time this is unsustainable and the consequences of low energy availability become apparent.

Unintentional under-fuelling is also common among athletes, particularly those who use active methods of travelling such as cycling or running to training. These athletes often underestimate the fuel required to replace energy spent during these journeys. There may be athletes who fuel adequately over the course of a day but who have energy deficits at certain points within the day (e.g. exercising before breakfast) and this can contribute to low energy availability (8). Carbohydrate availability around training seems to be of particular importance, especially when recovering from RED-S. Fasted sessions should be strongly discouraged. Emphasis in endurance training is on fuelling before, during and after sessions. The intensity of sessions should also be reduced during a phased return to training. The return to training and increase in activity should progress concurrently with physiological recovery and progress in therapy. This emphasises the importance of a multidisciplinary approach and collaboration between athlete, coach and the clinical team (1).

Not all athletes who suffer from RED-S have a low BMI or disordered eating (9). Many athletes struggle to understand that they are suffering from low energy availability if they are not losing weight. In a chronic low-energy state, the body prioritises movement over biological function, leading to down-regulation of metabolic rate to preserve energy.

RED-S, OTS, Disordered Eating and Eating Disorders

There is often significant overlap between these conditions, all of which affect both health and performance.

- OTS is a state of maladaptation due to excessive training load without adequate recovery to adapt to training. Performance will decline even with adequate fuelling
- Under-fuelling will cause performance decline even in cases where training load is appropriate
- Under-fuelling can be unintentional or the result of disordered eating or an eating disorder
- Athletes who both under-fuel and overtrain are at highest risk of developing RED-S

Q3) B

The eating and training behaviours of athletes with RED-S can be a coping strategy for an underlying anxiety (which may or may not be related to their sport) and this relationship can also be found in eating disorders (10). Athletes may assign disproportionate importance to their body shape and success in sport. Whether or not the athlete's eating and training behaviours were initially driven by performance enhancement, they may reach a stage where they are a self-protective mechanism to avoid anxiety and distress. Engaging athletes in therapy and changing their behaviour can therefore be extremely challenging.

Common drivers of both under-fuelling and overtraining behaviours either in isolation or in combination are an inability to manage expectation (particularly in junior athletes) and perfectionism. Perfectionism is seen as desirable in sport and is therefore a common personality trait in athletes (11). However, 'excessive conscientiousness', 'rigidity' and a 'preoccupation with details' are all considered pathological under different circumstances and have been associated with an increased risk of eating disorders, OTS and exercise dependence (12,13,14,15).

It may be difficult to convince athletes that they are not fuelling adequately if they are not losing weight. Providing athletes with objective evidence in the form of blood tests can help them to gain insight into their condition (and that the body's compensatory shutting down of particular functions may be enough to prevent weight loss but is causing long-term harm in order to preserve energy).

CBT can bring about resumption of ovulatory menstrual cycles and neuroendocrine recovery in athletes with menstrual disturbances associated with RED-S (16,17,18). In a self-reported retrospective study, it was found that the two factors that most commonly facilitated recovery in female collegiate athletes with eating disorders were motivation to return to sport and a shifting of values and beliefs (19). Return to sport can motivate recovery even in those whose pathological behaviours are driven by performance (20). CBT can be effective in helping an athlete to understand and address underlying anxiety/low self-esteem, personality traits contributing to their behaviour (e.g. perfectionism), and to challenge fixed beliefs around body shape/eating and training behaviours and performance. By helping an athlete to consider both the perceived benefits and costs of their eating disorder, motivational interviewing can also be an effective therapeutic tool (21,22).

Q4)   A, C, D

The features of exercise addiction are similar to those of substance use disorders and include the negative effects as the addiction progresses to affect many areas of life including relationships and emotional wellbeing (23,24,25).

As with B, athletes will often say that their training and attitude is 'normal' for elite level competitors. There is overlap between athletic training and exercise addiction. For example, athletic training impacts on social life and other commitments; athletes spend a large proportion of time training and they may experience withdrawal phenomena when they stop (anhedonia, anxiety, irritability and disturbed sleep). However, athletes are able to control their time spent exercising and stop when they complete what they set out to do or when ill or injured. In exercise addiction the behaviour is continued despite its harmful consequences and it is increasingly difficult not to surpass the intended duration/intensity/frequency of training.

While training is initially driven by the positive reinforcement of progress and achieving goals, over time negative reinforcement may appear with training driven by the desire to avoid negative outcomes such as a performance plateau. If this happens (as is common in the transition from junior to senior participation) athletes may begin to overtrain and are more likely to develop exercise addiction.

The presentation of exercise addiction can overlap with OTS and RED-S and all may present with overuse injuries or endocrine disturbances. A careful history is required exploring the athlete's attitude and motivation for training alongside the nature of training (frequency, intensity and duration) with particular attention to any deviations from the prescribed training plan. It is possible to suffer from exercise addiction and fuel adequately (primary exercise addiction) but the compulsive exercise seen in those with eating disorders (secondary exercise addiction) is driven by the need to lose weight. This type of secondary addiction is associated with a more severe form of RED-S with more symptoms and more significant health consequences.

A risk factor for exercise addiction is starting to exercise with the goal of alleviating distress rather than as a pursuit in itself (26). So while there are mental (and physical) health benefits from exercise, those who use exercise as the sole coping strategy for unpleasant experiences or to improve their self-esteem are more at risk of developing exercise addiction (27). Other risk factors include choice of sport, with runners and triathletes at higher risk (23). Finally, there are genetic and psychological contributions to the risk of developing addictions in general that also increase the risk of a specific exercise addiction.

The treatment of exercise addiction can follow the same approach as other forms of addiction. For example, motivational interviewing to help an athlete move through the stages of behavioural change, CBT with the goal of introducing more flexibility to an exercise regime and other psychological skills to manage distress rather than relying solely on exercise. During the process of recovery it is beneficial for athletes to learn the differences between pain and fatigue and healthy or unhealthy motivators. Healthy motivators may include exploring one's capabilities and focusing on process-orientated goals: 'I am going to try out a new tactic in this race to add to my skill set', 'As long as I do my best I will be happy'. Whereas unhealthy motivators include: 'I need to run fast because then I will get praise', 'I have to go for a run today even though I feel ill because that is what is on my training schedule'.

Q 5) False

Return to play (RTP) during recovery from RED-S is a complicated process that needs to be managed on an individualised basis. However, there are important general principles and when assessing an athlete for returning to training it is important to take into consideration clinical examination, blood test results, nutritional assessment and progression/resolution of symptoms. Input from a clinical psychologist/psychiatrist or other therapist where appropriate and involvement of the coach when discussing appropriate training load and intensity (7,28) will also aid the decision. For junior athletes who still live in the family home, it is highly desirable for parents or guardians to engage in the process of recovery.

A risk stratification and management tool is now widely used to assess the risks associated with an athlete's RTP (7). This was designed for those athletes who suffer from disordered eating or clinical eating disorders specifically. The tool classifies athletes as low, medium and high risk for RTS. B scored as follows: 2 points for having less than 6 periods in the past 12 months, 1 point for a DEXA scan Z score between -1 and -2, and 2 points for having had 2 or more stress fractures or stress responses. Her total score was 5, which put her in the moderate category where provisional or limited clearance was recommended for her RTP.

Written contracts are used for some athletes to outline how the athlete should expect to be assessed by the multidisciplinary team (MDT) and what treatment targets are required for their continued safe participation in sport. It has been suggested that a signed written contract is required for those in moderate- and high-risk groups (7). For those within high-risk categories, RTP is not recommended and some athletes may not achieve required modifications in their risk stratification plan that enables this. Contracts clearly outline what is required for the athlete's recovery and the benefits and consequences associated with meeting/not meeting the requirements (1,7). During this period, the athlete will receive support from the MDT at an agreed frequency with agreed targets. If an athlete is compliant with their tailored treatment plan and continues to progress then their activity levels can continue and increase as appropriate. If the athlete is not compliant or able to maintain progress then their activity level may have to be reduced or their medical clearance to participate may need to be reviewed. Psychological recovery is likely to take longer than physical recovery, and returning to training may trigger pathological training and eating behaviours. It is therefore important to re-evaluate the appropriateness of RTP after training resumes and appreciate that medical clearance may not be a permanent state.

Summary of the Chapter and the Topics Covered

- The presence of RED-S, disordered eating and exercise addiction within adult, elite sport
- Issues specific to the female athlete
- OTS in endurance sport
- Psychotherapy for eating disorders
- Exercise as a treatment for mental illness

References

1. Mountjoy M, Sundgot-Borgen J, Burke L, Carter S, Constantini N, Lebrun C, et al. The IOC consensus statement: Beyond the Female Athlete Triad-Relative Energy Deficiency in Sport (RED-S). *Br J Sports Med*. 2014;48(7):491–7. Available from: http://bjsm.bmj.com/content/48/7/491 .abstract

2. American Psychiatric Association. *Diagnostic and Statistical Manual of Mental Disorders (DSM-5)*. 5th edition. Washington, DC: American Psychiatric Publishing; 2013 [cited 2018 Jun 29]. 1–947. Available from: www.appi.org/Course/Boo k/Subscription/JournalSubscription/id-332 2/Diagnostic_and_Statistical_Manual_of_ Mental_Disorders_%28DSM-5®%29

3. Frisch RE. Body fat, puberty and fertility. *Biol Rev Camb Philos Soc*. 1984;59 (2):161–88.

4. Loucks AB. Energy balance and body composition in sports and exercise. In: *Journal of Sports Sciences*. 2004. 1–14.

5. Mountjoy M, Sundgot-Borgen JK, Burke LM, Ackerman KE, Blauwet C, Constantini N, et al. IOC consensus statement on relative energy deficiency in sport (RED-S): 2018 update. *Br J Sports Med*. 2018;52(11):687–97.

6. Gordon CM, Ackerman KE, Berga SL, Kaplan JR, Mastorakos G, Misra M, et al. Functional hypothalamic amenorrhea: An endocrine society clinical practice guideline. *J Clin Endocrinol Metab*. 2017;102 (5):1413–39.

7. Joy E, Kussman A, Nattiv A. Update on eating disorders in athletes: A comprehensive narrative review with a focus on clinical assessment and management. *Br J Sports Med*. 2016;50 (3):154–62. Available from: http://bjsm .bmj.com/lookup/doi/10.1136 /bjsports-2015–095735

8. Fahrenholtz IL, Sjödin A, Benardot D, Tornberg B, Skouby S, Faber J, et al. Within-day energy deficiency and reproductive function in female endurance athletes. *Scand J Med Sci Sport*. 2018;28 (3):1139–46.

9. Melin A, Tornberg B, Skouby S, Møller SS, Sundgot-Borgen J, Faber J, et al. Energy availability and the female athlete triad in elite endurance athletes. *Scand J Med Sci Sport*. 2015;25(5):610–22.

10. Abbate-Daga F, Delsedime, N, De-Bacco, C, Fassino, SGA. *Resistance to treatment and change in anorexia nervosa [corrected]: a clinical overview.[Erratum appears in BMC Psychiatry. 2014; 14:62]. BMC Psychiatry*. 2013 [cited 2019 Dec 7];13:294. Available from: http://ovidsp.ovid.com/ov idweb.cgi?T=JS&CSC=Y&NEWS=N&PA GE=fulltext&D=prem&AN=24199620; htt p://dc8qa4cy3 n.search.serialssolutions.co m/?url_ver=Z39.88–2004&rft_val_fm t=info:ofi/fmt:kev:mtx:journal&rfr_i d=info:sid/Ovid:prem&rft.genre=arti cle&rft_id=info:doi/

11. Haase AM, Prapavessis H, Glynn Owens R. Perfectionism, social physique anxiety and disordered eating: A comparison of male and female elite athletes. *Psychol Sport Exerc*. 2002;3(3):209–22.

12. WHO. *International Statistical Classification of Diseases and Related Health Problems: 10th revision*. World Health Organization. 2011.

13. Madigan DJ, Stoeber J, Passfield L. Perfectionism and training distress in junior athletes: A longitudinal

investigation. *J Sports Sci.* 2017;35 (5):470–5.

14. Forsberg S, Lock J. The relationship between perfectionism, eating disorders and athletes: A review. *Minerva Pediatr.* 2006;58(6):525–36.

15. Downs DS, Hausenblas HA, Nigg CR. Factorial validity and psychometric examination of the exercise dependence scale-revised. *Meas Phys Educ Exerc Sci.* 2004;8(4):183–201.

16. Arends JC, Cheung M-YC, Barrack MT, Nattiv A. Restoration of menses with nonpharmacologic therapy in college athletes With menstrual disturbances: A 5-year retrospective study. *Int J Sport Nutr Exerc Metab.* 2012 [cited 2019 Dec 7];22 (2):98–108. Available from: http://connec tion.ebscohost.com/c/articles/73445467/re storation-menses-nonpharmacologic-therapy-college-athletes-menstrual-disturbances-5-year-retrospective-study

17. Berga SL, Marcus MD, Loucks TL, Hlastala S, Ringham R, Krohn MA. Recovery of ovarian activity in women with functional hypothalamic amenorrhea who were treated with cognitive behavior therapy. *Fertil Steril.* 2003 [cited 2019 Dec 7];80(4):976–81. Available from: www .ncbi.nlm.nih.gov/pubmed/14556820

18. Michopoulos V, Mancini F, Loucks TL, Berga SL. Neuroendocrine recovery initiated by cognitive behavioral therapy in women with functional hypothalamic amenorrhea: A randomized, controlled trial. *Fertil Steril.* 2013;99(7).

19. Arthur-Cameselle JN, Quatromoni PA. Eating disorders in collegiate female athletes: Factors that assist recovery. *Eat Disord.* 2014;22(1):50–61.

20. Papathomas A, Lavallee D. Self-starvation and the performance narrative in competitive sport. *Psychol Sport Exerc.* 2014;15(6):688–95. Available from: http://d x.doi.org/10.1016/j.psychsport.2013.10.014

21. Miller WR, Rollnick S. Motivational interviewing: Preparing people to change addictive behavior. Miller WR, Rollnick S,

eds. *Journal of Community and Applied Social Psychology.* 1st edition. New York, NY: Guilford Press; 1991 [cited 2019 Dec 7]. Available from: http://doi .wiley.com/10.1002/casp.2450020410

22. Woolsey CL, Mannion J, Williams RD, Steffen W, Aruguete MS, Evans MW, et al. Understanding emotional and binge eating: From sports training to tailgating. *The Sport Journal.* 2013 [cited 2019 Dec 7]. Available from: http://thesportjournal.org /article/understanding-emotional-and-binge-eating-from-sports-training-to-tailgating/

23. Hausenblas HA, Schreiber K, Smoliga JM. Addiction to exercise. *BMJ.* 2017; 26 (357):1745.

24. Griffiths MD, Szabo A, Terry A. The exercise addiction inventory: A quick and easy screening tool for health practitioners. *Br J Sports Med.* 2005;39(6).

25. Freimuth M, Moniz S, Kim SR. Clarifying exercise addiction: Differential diagnosis, co-occurring disorders, and phases of addiction. *Int J Environ Res Public Health.* 2011;8(10):4069–81.

26. Thornton EW, Scott SE. Motivation in the committed runner: Correlations between self-report scales and behaviour. *Health Promot Int.* 1995 [cited 2019 Dec 7];10 (3):177–84. Available from: https://aca demic.oup.com/heapro/article-lookup/do i/10.1093/heapro/10.3.177

27. Scully D, Kremer J, Meade M, Graham R, Dudgeon K. Physical exercise and psychological well being: A critical review. *Br J Sports Med.* 1998;32 (2):111–20.

28. De Souza MJ, Nattiv A, Joy E, Misra M, Williams NI, Mallinson RJ, et al. Female athlete triad coalition consensus statement on treatment and return to play of the female athlete triad: 1st international conference held in San Francisco, California, May 2012 and 2nd international conference held in Indianapolis, Indiana, M. *Br J Sports Med.* 2014;48(4):289.

Chapter 3

Boxing: Low Mood and Gambling

Allan Johnston and Marwan Al-Dawoud
Athlete expert advisor: Cyrus Pattinson

Sports psychiatrists should be familiar with the associations related to contact sport head injuries in boxing and increased risk of neuropsychiatric sequelae. However, similar to the general population, boxers can also experience mood disorders such as depression and other psychiatric co-morbidities. These may include anxiety disorders, personality disorders and addictions (1) such as gambling disorder. Prevalence studies suggest higher rates of gambling problems among athletes than the general population (2). Common risks including suicide or self-harm must also be assessed. Psychiatric consultations should determine the type and severity of mood disorder alongside the impact of any co-morbid conditions. A psychiatrist needs to make a thorough assessment of core mental health conditions while simultaneously considering a range of differential diagnoses and co-morbidities to ensure a holistic, biopsychosocial care plan can be implemented.

Background

DB is a 24-year-old, Caucasian middleweight boxer with a national Olympic team's world-class programme. As a consequence of his boxing career he had sustained several minor concussions and been assessed at a regional concussion clinic by a consultant neurologist.

During the working week he used to train with the Olympic team at their base living in 'team digs' and at weekends travelled home to his girlfriend, Emily, and his family, who lived in a rural village. At times he felt isolated in a city environment and had found it hard to make friends with his boxing peers, who seemed different from him. When at home, D lived with his girlfriend, Emily, in a rented townhouse and also saw his family who lived nearby. When in digs, he had less structure and support and as a result his pattern of eating and sleeping would become less regular. With few friends and no structure to his free time D had taken to going to a local casino as a 'pick me up' on an evening after sparring.

Over the last three months his boxing coaches had become concerned at his loss of motivation and enjoyment for his sport. Initially he had started to arrive late at the gym, appearing tired, and on a couple of occasions on the verge of tears. He had since missed a team trip to Thailand reporting that he 'didn't feel right to go'. He had gained weight and struggled to make the weight limit for his next fight. His coaches requested the team doctor to speak to him. After this consultation he agreed to the team doctor making a referral to a sports psychiatrist. The notes of the consultation with the sports psychiatrist are outlined below:

Presenting Complaint

'I'm just not enjoying my boxing like I used to, maybe this life is not for me anymore.'

History of Presenting Complaint

D reported a six-month history of low mood and increased, out-of-character tiredness following routine boxing training sessions. He continued to attend the majority of gym and sparring sessions although without the same enjoyment or enthusiasm. Despite feeling tired, the quality of his sleep was worse with a more irregular pattern. When in team digs he would not sleep until around midnight but also reported waking earlier than usual, at around 5am. On occasions when he would stay later in the casino trying to 'chase losses' he would not get to bed until 3am. At weekends back at home he tried to catch up on sleep, which frustrated his girlfriend given their limited time together.

D's appetite had altered in that he could not motivate himself to cook healthy meals as he previously had done and instead would 'eat crap', choosing take-away food or the free food provided to him by the casino as a 'VIP guest'. He had gained 5kg in weight and was currently 82kg. He would usually be around 77kg and found it increasingly difficult to make the 75kg weight limit for his middleweight classification. The team nutritionist had provided personalised advice but he had found it difficult to implement it. Previously he enjoyed reading books before bed, particularly about his boxing heroes Nigel Benn and Chris Eubank. He had now fallen out of this habit due to frustration related to his inability to concentrate while reading each page.

When in camp at the national centre he tried to focus on his boxing but had few friends in whom he could confide. He felt 'different to these big-city kids' and acknowledged that he used to make more of an effort to spend time with his peers. When at home D was something of a well-known local celebrity and as a result had felt reluctant discussing his recent problems with family or friends. In many ways he was 'living the dream lifestyle of his schooldays', but the reality was that of relative isolation in a big city far from home, away from his real support network of family and friends. His isolation was coupled with strong perfectionistic personality traits and a high internal locus of control (the degree to which people believe that they should have control over the outcome of events in their lives) meaning that even when the opportunity arose to seek support he was inhibited from doing so.

Following feelings of isolation, D started to get out of his digs and began to visit his local casino. He would initially spend a maximum of £20 and felt that he was unaffected by wins or losses. However, on one occasion around six months previously, he had won a significant four-figure sum. His gambling had since increased in terms of frequency of visits and the amount that he spent. Over recent weeks he was gambling up to four days per week and had spent increasing quantities of up to £3,000 per day. Also, being recognised by casino staff as an Olympic boxer and high spender, he was soon upgraded to 'VIP guest' status, meaning that he was given exclusive access to certain roulette tables and was provided with free food and drinks all night. Over time, his interests narrowed to that of gambling and boxing only.

D had generated a degree of debt as a result of his gambling. This was initially funded by his income and later by the savings he intended to use to purchase a house with his girlfriend. Over the last month he had needed to ask a boxing peer, Danny, to lend him money, reporting (untruthfully) that a sponsor had not paid on time. He now owed Danny £50,000.

He recognised gambling had been harmful for his physical health affecting his sleep and energy levels in the gym. He had been berating himself for letting his girlfriend and everyone else down. He was unhappy at his deceit with Danny, which resulted in worsening his low self-esteem. He was unable to speak to Emily about this and had become 'snappy' with her.

He described features of dependency including cravings for gambling, having frequent thoughts of gambling and that these took up increasing quantities of his time. He presented with 'primacy' as gambling took precedence over other important factors in his life including his boxing career. Gambling had caused him to arrive late for training and he had at times been distracted in training by thoughts preoccupied with his next gambling spree. The frequency of his casino visits and the amount he spent each time had both increased significantly. He had contemplated cutting back on his gambling but was unable to action these genuine intentions.

He felt that life was becoming 'too much' and wished he could 'escape' from the situation. There were no reported substance addictions or other behavioural addictions related to pornography, gaming or problematic internet use. He possessed several well-known social media accounts but felt that he used them in a moderate, controlled manner.

Past Psychiatric History

Prior to this episode D had no history of mental illness. Three years ago he reported feeling lonely and unhappy for some weeks after separating from his ex-partner, Kate, but had not required any treatment and this resolved with support from his friends. No prior periods of elevated mood were described.

Family History

D disclosed that his mother suffered from recurrent depression and had taken eight courses of antidepressant medication. She was currently under the care of her local Community Mental Health Team. He denied his older sister possessing any reported mental health problems. He suspected that his maternal grandmother also had depression but the family never spoke about this in his presence.

Past Medical History

D had a superior labral anterior-to-posterior tear of the right shoulder that was surgically repaired three years ago.

A 'boxer's' fracture of the fifth metacarpal (MCP) on the right side one year ago was conservatively managed.

D had had three concussions over the past two years for which he had seen a concussion specialist. Serial MRI brain scans have not revealed any acute intracranial pathology such as traumatic bleeds or lobar atrophy (deemed 'normal') and he had successfully returned to competition in line with standard graded return to perform protocols on each occasion.

Medication History

No known drug allergies, D had never been prescribed any psychiatric medication.

Tramadol 100mg when required (PRN) for analgesia, usually one or two tablets on fight night and during the week if he was experiencing any pain.

D took protein, creatine and vitamin supplements on a daily, regimented basis.

Social History

D lived with his girlfriend and her 12-year-old son, Kade, in a rented property. He had a 7-year-old daughter, Bella, who lived with his ex-partner, Kate, a few hours' drive away. He saw his daughter once or twice a month. During the week he was resident in a single flat alone as part of shared 'digs' with his boxing peers but did not feel able to socialise with them. His parents were separated but both still lived in the same small rural village, two hours away from Manchester. D was close to his girlfriend's family. They lived nearby and he saw them most weekends.

Until recently, D denied possessing any reported financial problems, although he now owed his friend £50,000. His current boxing salary from his national governing body was no longer enough to meet his problematic gambling needs and he was unsure how he could pay his friend back. He admitted to once taking cocaine after a big fight when encouraged by a friend but had not repeated this. He wondered if he was 'easily led' by peer pressure. He was a non-smoker and denied any other illicit drug use. He would previously have avoided alcohol but had started to consume up to four units of lager a night, every time he visited the casino, up to four times a week.

Personal History

D denied any reported complications at birth and achieved normal childhood developmental milestones. He enjoyed attending school and was popular within his year, particularly excelling at physical education. His parents separated when he was 13 years old. He recalled hearing frequent arguments and occasional fights through the walls of his bedroom at night. His mother developed depression after the separation and still struggled with her mental health. He remained close to his mother and always visited her when back home. His sister lived close by although they had fallen out when their parents got divorced; she decided to go to live with their dad and D opted to stay to look after their mum.

During his teenage years, he threw himself into boxing with a local amateur club, partly as escapism from his stressful home environment. He would sometimes miss schoolwork to attend the boxing gym instead. He did not possess any educational qualifications or any vocational training. At the age of 18, he moved away from his family home to train with the national team and was supported in his boxing career through the central funding programme.

D had had two long-term heterosexual relationships. He met his first girlfriend, Kate, at school when they were both 15 years old. There was an unplanned pregnancy two years later, which resulted in the birth of his daughter, Bella. They separated shortly afterwards when D trained away from home and Kate moved with Bella to another city three hours away. His current girlfriend, Emily, was 28 years old and lived in northwest England with D and her son, Kade, aged 12 and from a previous relationship.

Pre-Morbid Personality

D described himself previously as 'quietly confident'. He tended to keep himself to himself but admitted to sometimes letting emotions get the better of him. More recently he had taken to punching the walls to let out his pent-up anger.

Forensic History

Six months ago he had been arrested and subsequently charged with actual bodily harm. He had lost some money at the local casino and was involved in an altercation with the casino security staff. His charge involved a fine and a community order. He denied any history of sexual misconduct or drug-related offences.

Collateral History

He refused consent for a collateral history to be obtained from family members although reported that his girlfriend had become worried about him and might wish to speak to his clinicians in future. D had instantly refused consent for his coaching team to be contacted regarding his recent behaviour and mental health.

Mental State Examination

D presented as a 24-year-old Caucasian male. He was well-kempt, wearing a baseball cap, designer t-shirt and skinny jeans. He had a tattoo on his left arm that was mostly covered by his t-shirt and the name of his daughter tattooed on the inside of his right forearm. His interaction was guarded initially, but he became more open as the conversation progressed. He demonstrated eye contact within the normal range throughout. His speech was normal in rate, tone and volume. His mood was subjectively and objectively low. He became tearful when discussing his relationship with his daughter, as he wanted to see her more and be a better dad, but was frustrated that he was not 'allowed to'. There were no abnormalities of thought form, flow or content. His perceptions were normal. He was fully orientated and scored 30/30 on Mini Mental State Examination (MMSE). He had partial insight in that he recognised his mood was very low. He acknowledged that gambling had become problematic but reported that he could get this under control and was 'definitely not addicted'.

Risk Assessment

Self: D reported some thoughts that life was becoming 'too much' and wished he could 'escape' from his stress at times. He denied any recent specific thoughts of methods of self-harm or suicide but did sometimes wonder if he would be 'better off dead'. He denied any plans or intentions to harm himself. He had never self-harmed in the past.

Others: No expressed risks to others at present. D admitted that he had become increasingly 'grumpy and snappy' at home towards his girlfriend, Emily, but denied any domestic violence. There were no known child protection issues identified.

Protective factors: He possessed a good support network at home. He enjoyed time with his family. He was motivated to address his low mood symptoms and engage in professional support. He demonstrated some insight into his gambling problem and had recognised the harm it had caused.

Investigations

Scored 19 on PHQ-9 and 8 on GAD-7.

Bony deformity over fifth MCP. Restriction to full flexion and abduction of right shoulder.

Cholesterol mildly raised at 5.4 mmol/L, all other bloods normal.

A urinary drug screen (UDS) was mildly positive for opioids (consistent with his tramadol use) but otherwise negative.

Case Formulation

D presented as a 24-year-old male Olympic boxer. His experience of low mood along with biological symptoms of insomnia, anergia and anhedonia were compatible with a diagnosis of a depressive episode. Within the past six months his gambling had developed into a dependent pattern. His mother's recurrent depression and his maternal grandmother's possible depression suggested a hereditary predisposing risk.

In terms of precipitating factors he was isolated, had few friends to whom he could speak and his alcohol consumption had increased. Perpetuating his condition, his co-morbid gambling behaviour had induced a sense of low self-esteem, particularly when he reflected on his recent lying behaviour to access funds for his habit. There was a sense of stigma around speaking about mental illness both within his family and to his boxing peers. His perfectionistic personality traits caused him to feel that his depressed mood was evidence that he had 'somehow failed' and further prevented him from seeking help.

There was a bidirectional relationship between his depressed mood and gambling dependency. Initially, gambling provided a required 'pick me up' for his low mood but then his subsequent losses impacted on his self-esteem and mood and led to further self-criticism. His coaches had noticed a loss of enthusiasm and his usual high athletic standards had dropped. He was open to accessing professional mental health help. He was able to identify protective factors in his family support network.

Plan

- D was offered a range of treatment options addressing biological, psychological and social factors in his illness and situation and reflecting a biopsychosocial approach to formulation and treatment
- He was provided with sleep hygiene advice, in particular the importance of establishing a good sleep routine
- D was given information about antidepressant medication options. He was willing to consider this but had concerns about side effects and especially any effects on his training and boxing performance. It was agreed this could be re-explored at his follow up outpatient appointment
- Several psychotherapy approaches were discussed. A programme of psycho-education was recommended around his dependence on gambling and he was directed towards sources of online information. A simple motivational interviewing (MI) strategy was used, initially asking D to consider the pros and cons of gambling and its effects on his life. In consideration of his depressed mood a CBT approach was discussed, with initial work centering on cognitive errors or biases in his self-concept and self-esteem

- His current relationships were explored. It was suggested that it might help if he spoke more openly to family and friends about his recent difficulties
- D was given information on a local gambling peer support group. He felt this would be helpful but was fearful he would be recognised by other members attending these groups
- D did not consent to a medical letter being sent to the team doctor or coach but agreed to consider this prior to his next appointment
- He was offered a further follow up at the sports psychiatry clinic in two weeks time to review his progress with the above initial psychotherapy approaches. It was agreed that he could be referred on to the national gambling clinic in London, UK, if he required further expert MDT intervention (e.g. naltrexone medication)
- Given his vague, passive suicidal thoughts, he was offered an emergency crisis plan in case his suicidal ideation intensified. D was given a crisis phone number to contact if he became mentally unwell outside normal working hours. Also, he agreed to contact emergency services and attend an accident and emergency department (A&E) if in severe mental distress and acutely suicidal

Questions

Q 1 According to DSM-V criteria, what severity is D's depression? (Please choose one)
  A. Euthymic (normal) mood
  B. Mild
  C. Moderate
  D. Severe
  E. Manic

Q 2 According to the latest National Institute for Health and Care Excellence (NICE) guidelines, what would be the preferred treatment(s) for a depressive episode in the moderate to severe category such as experienced by D? (Please choose one)
  A. A psychological treatment alone, e.g. CBT
  B. Antidepressant medication alone, e.g. an antidepressant from the SSRI class (e.g. citalopram or fluoxetine)
  C. A combination of psychological treatment and antidepressant medication
  D. Electroconvulsive therapy (ECT)
  E. No treatment is necessary at present but follow-up should be offered to ensure the situation is resolving ('watchful waiting')

Q 3 Which of the following of D's behaviours meet the DSM-V criteria for a gambling disorder? (Please choose all that apply)
  A. Relies on others to provide money to relieve desperate financial situations caused by gambling
  B. Lies to conceal the extent of involvement with gambling
  C. Is restless or irritable when attempting to cut down or stop gambling
  D. Loss of interest in usual pleasurable activities as a result of gambling
  E. Needs to gamble increasing amounts of money in order to achieve the desired excitement

Q 4 D's team doctor calls you as his sports psychiatrist after this first appointment and requests the diagnosis and treatment plan. How do you respond?
  A. Discuss diagnosis but not treatment
  B. Discuss the treatment but not diagnosis
  C. Tell the team doctor you cannot disclose any information without gaining consent from D
  D. Find out what the team doctor knows, and only elaborate on information which is already known to him
  E. Without going into specifics, give the team doctor vague information about D's diagnosis, treatment and risk

Q 5 CBT is the most effective form of psychological intervention for problem gambling. (True or False?)

Answers

Q 1) C

The fifth edition of the Diagnostic and Statistical Manual of Mental Disorders, DSM-V (1), describes the principal features of major depressive disorder (MDD) and in addition specifies severity criteria. Nine symptom groups are described beginning with low mood and significantly reduced interest/pleasure as central features. In addition, the patient may experience any of seven additional symptoms. These are tiredness/fatigue, significant weight changes (increased or reduced weight), significant sleep disturbance (reduced or increased sleep), psychomotor changes (agitation or retardation), excessive thoughts of guilt or worthlessness, impaired concentration/indecision and finally thoughts/plans of death or suicide.

Five or more symptoms must be present for at least two weeks and on nearly every day with significant impairment in function (e.g. socially or at work) to make a diagnosis of MDD. The disorder is described as mild if there are just enough symptoms to make the diagnosis and if functional impairment is minimal and distress manageable. It is described as severe if almost all the symptoms are present and causing major distress and functional impairment. Psychotic symptoms may be seen if the disorder is very severe and if present are usually 'mood congruent', i.e. reflecting the sufferer's severely depressed mood state. Examples might include delusions of guilt or poverty or self-critical auditory hallucinations.

A diagnosis of persistent depressive disorder or dysthymia may be made if there are relatively few (two or more) symptoms alongside depressed mood but if these have been endured for two years or more.

The International Classification of Diseases (ICD10) (2) is another internationally recognised diagnostic manual for standardising the diagnosis of health conditions and describes broadly comparable criteria. In a typical depressive episode the patient experiences symptoms of low mood, reduced energy, decreased activity and anhedonia (diminished pleasure in activities). Additional features include impaired concentration, tiredness, low self-esteem and self-confidence, and ideas of guilt or worthlessness. 'Somatic' symptoms may be experienced including waking early in the morning, mood lowest in the morning (diurnal mood variation), psychomotor changes of retardation or agitation, loss of appetite, weight loss and reduced libido. The condition would be described as mild if only two to three symptoms are present with minimal distress or impairment, moderate if four or more and severe if most symptoms are seen alongside marked distress or impairment. Both classificatory systems further sub-classify depressive disorders into single episode or recurrent episodes.

Another important consideration is that there must have been no previous episodes of mania or hypomania. The presence of either would instead point to a diagnosis of bipolar affective disorder. It is important not to miss this diagnosis as bipolar depressive episodes do not respond as well to conventional antidepressant medication. Also antidepressant prescriptions in bipolar affective disorder can even induce difficult-to-treat manic or mixed affective episodes (3). Symptoms of mania and hypomania usually consist of an elevation of mood with increased energy and activity. Other symptoms include a reduced need for sleep, increased appetite and reduced concentration. The mental state examination may reveal clothing which is colourful or inappropriate for the season, periods of agitation or irritability, pressure of speech (rapid speech rate) or flight of ideas (rapidly changing flow of thoughts). In severe episodes there may be mood-congruent psychotic symptoms such as grandiose delusions or hallucinations (1,2).

In mania the functional impairment is marked but in hypomania this is less so, such that the patient may not have presented for medical attention. Therefore the vigilant clinician will gently enquire and screen all patients presenting for the first time with depression for prior episodes of hypomania and mania (4). The diagnosis can be more difficult to establish in elite athletes where overactivity may be harder to spot in those who are training intensely or where intense exercise may provide an outlet for the excess energy of mood disturbance (5,6). An additional complication is that some substances occasionally misused by athletes such as stimulants and anabolic androgenic steroids, may induce hypomanic symptoms (7,8).

In D's case there was no history of substance misuse and toxicology was negative. He had no other medical or psychiatric condition that might explain his depressive symptoms and no history of mood elevation (although a collateral history would help to verify this). He possessed a sufficiently broad range of symptoms that would qualify as severe although his functional impairment and distress were not deemed to be in the severe range.

Q 2) C

The NICE Guidance for Depression (9) is widely used in the UK and beyond. Treatments are recommended based on the severity of the episode. In moderate to severe depression, a combination of antidepressant medication and a high-intensity psychological intervention is recommended.

In cases of mild to moderate depression, sole antidepressant medication or a high-intensity, 1:1 psychological intervention tend to be offered. Medication options tend to be first-line SSRIs, whereas psychological interventions include CBT, interpersonal therapy (IPT), behavioural activation or couples' therapy. Also, the use of programmed physical activity and group exercise should not be overlooked, particularly in the elderly population.

The tolerability and safety of antidepressant medication is an important consideration when prescribing for athletes (10). Side effects that could affect performance include sedation, weight gain and cardiac side effects (10). While there are no research studies that have been conducted in athlete-specific populations expert opinion has favoured sertraline (11) and fluoxetine (12) among the SSRI class.

ECT is reserved for severe, treatment-resistant depression and where delay to treatment could be life-threatening for the patient (e.g. those in depressed stupor whose physical health has become unstable).

Q 3)   A, B, C and E

The Diagnostic and Statistical Manual for Mental Illness (DSM-V) (1) describes the criteria for gambling disorder. To diagnose a disorder, gambling behaviour should have led to significant distress or impairment during the previous 12 months and should not be the consequence of another condition such as mania in bipolar disorder.

Nine clinical features are described and at least four must be present to make a diagnosis. The sufferer typically has to gamble increasing amounts to achieve the same level of excitement (tolerance). They may be restless or irritable when trying to cut down or stop (withdrawal). They may already have made several attempts to reduce or stop gambling. They might describe persistent/dominant thoughts of gambling including mentally going over previous gambling and planning future gambling (preoccupation). Gambling when feeling anxious, depressed or otherwise distressed is often seen. Sufferers will often gamble shortly after a loss in order to get even again. They may conceal or minimise the extent of their gambling. Relationships, jobs and education/career opportunities may be compromised by gambling. Finally the gambler may become reliant on family, friends and acquaintances to supply money to pay off debts.

A gambling disorder is classified mild if four to five criteria are met, moderate if six to seven criteria are met and severe if eight to nine criteria are present.

Q 4)   C

While it can often be helpful to share necessary information about a patient's treatment and care with others involved in that care, disclosures to third parties (as in this case) should only be made with the patient's consent and only information relevant to the request should be disclosed (not the whole patient record: www.gmc-uk.org/ethical-guidance/ethical-guidance-for-doctors/confidentiality).

Confidentiality is for privacy not secrecy and is a vital part of the doctor–patient relationship. The sporting environment provides a unique setting in which to test this. Clinicians' obligations, physical environments, demands from coaching staff and practice and policy contexts all contribute to the pressure on the doctor's duty of confidentiality(13). In light of these challenges, there are several areas to consider:

- **Roles:** make a clear separation of the sports medicine role and encourage athletes to have their own general practitioner
- **Clarity:** clinicians, coaching staff and athletes should be fully aware of the healthcare systems in which they are operating
- **Contracts:** sports doctors should consider having formal contracts, which may help to reduce the conflict between occupational expectations and medical ethical principles

- **Education:** physicians should keep themselves up to date on current ethical standards. Governing bodies can develop and disseminate models of good practice and promote learning through continuing professional development
- **Facilities:** medical and consultation facilities should be provided which safeguard patient privacy

Q 5) False

There are currently no NICE guidelines for the treatment of gambling in the UK, which like many other countries refers to the 2011 Australian National Health and Medical Research Council guidelines (14).

CBT seems more effective than no intervention but there is insufficient evidence to determine whether it is superior to other psychological treatments. CBT should be delivered by CBT-trained professionals and the therapy should be manual-guided.

MI and motivational enhancement therapy also seem to be more effective than no treatment and, once again, should be delivered by a trained clinician with a manualised structure. Practitioner-delivered treatment interventions seem more effective than self-help groups and the evidence for group interventions is currently limited.

Further studies are needed to assess whether there is evidence for inpatient treatment. It is also unclear whether abstinence-based programmes are more effective than those without a total abstinence goal and more research is required here, too. However, as with alcohol dependence it is appropriate to continue to work with those who are not currently committed to abstinence rather than deny access to treatment.

On review of medication options, naltrexone can be used to reduce gambling severity but should be prescribed by an experienced practitioner with consideration of contraindications such as concurrent opiate use. Antidepressant medication cannot be recommended as there is no evidence that this improves gambling outcomes. Standard antidepressant treatments such as SSRIs should be reserved for when there is a co-morbid depressive disorder or other condition requiring this treatment.

The Royal College of Psychiatrists has made a series of recommendations on problem gambling covering the need for further research, better services, improved access to treatments, developing treatment guidelines and training in problem gambling. These are available from: www.rcpsych.ac.uk/members/your-faculties/addictions-psychiatry/news-and-resources. Firstly, the College recommends that randomised controlled treatment trials should be conducted in the UK as gambling-related harm, gambling definitions, the use of gambling-related products and treatment provision differ so widely from country to country. Secondly, gambling disorder is a mental disorder with significant levels of harm to individuals and society, and treatment services should have parity with other mental disorders, in particular other addictions. Thirdly, naltrexone is the treatment intervention of choice for treatment-resistant gambling and should be available for affected patients. Fourthly, NICE guidelines are required to address a common problem that has not been sufficiently prioritised by the NHS. Finally, training in problem gambling should be included in medical student and postgraduate psychiatry training curriculum.

Summary of the Chapter and the Topics Covered

- The presentation of a depressive episode in elite sport
- Gambling disorder as a common co-morbidity
- A biopsychosocial approach to clinical care
- Confidentiality and the duties of a sports physician
- Clinical approaches to managing gambling disorders

References

1. American Psychiatric Association. *Diagnostic and Statistical Manual of Mental Disorders (DSM-5).* 5th ed. Washington, DC: American Psychiatric Publishing; 2013 [cited 2018 Jun 29]. 1–947. Available from: www.appi.org/Course/Book/Subscription/JournalSubscription/id-3322/Diagnostic_and_Statistical_Manual_of_Mental_Disorders_%28DSM-5®%29

2. World Health Organization. *International Statistical Classification of Diseases and Related Health Problems – 10th Revision.* World Health Organization. 2011.

3. Goldberg JF, Truman CJ. Antidepressant-induced mania: An overview of current controversies. *Bipolar Disord.* 2003;5 (6):407–20.

4. Goodwin GM, Haddad PM, Ferrier IN, Aronson JK, Barnes TRH, Cipriani A, et al. Evidence-based guidelines for treating bipolar disorder: Revised third edition recommendations from the British Association for Psychopharmacology. *J Psychopharmacol.* 2016;30(6):495–553.

5. Markser V, Currie A, McAllister-Williams RH. Mood disorders. In: Currie A, Owen B, editors. *Sports Psychiatry.* Oxford: Oxford University Press; 2016. p. 31–51.

6. Currie A, Gorczynski P, Rice SM, Purcell R, McAllister-Williams RH, Hitchcock ME, et al. Bipolar and psychotic disorders in elite athletes: A narrative review. *Br J Sports Med.* 2019 May 16 [cited 2019 May 17]; bjsports-2019–100685. Available from: http://bjsm.bmj.com/lookup/doi/10.1136/bjsports-2019–100685

7. Reardon C, Creado S. Drug abuse in athletes. *Substance Abuse and Rehabilitation.* 2014;(5):95–105. Available from: www.dovepress.com/drug-abuse-in-athletes-peer-reviewed-article-SAR

8. Baron DA, Reardon CL, Baron SH. Doping in sport. In: Baron DA, Reardon CL, Baron SH, eds. *Clinical Sports Psychiatry: An International Perspective.* 1st edition. Oxford: John Wiley & Sons; 2013 [cited 2017 Dec 12]. p. 21–32. Available from: http://doi.wiley.com/10.1002/9781118404904.ch3

9. National Institute for Health and Care Excellence. *Depression in Adults: Recognition and Management.* Clinical guideline CG90. [cited 2016 Feb 19]; Available from: www.nice.org.uk/guidance/cg90

10. Reardon CL, Hainline B, Aron CM, Baron D, Baum AL, Bindra A, et al. Mental health in elite athletes: International Olympic Committee consensus statement (2019). *Br J Sports Med.* 2019 Jun 1 [cited 2019 May 29];53(11):667–99. Available from: www.ncbi.nlm.nih.gov/pubmed/31097450

11. Johnston A, McAllister-Williams RH. Psychotropic drug prescribing. In: Currie A, Owen B, eds. *Sports Psychiatry.* 1st edition. Oxford: Oxford University Press; 2016. p. 133–43.

12. Reardon CL, Creado S. Psychiatric medication preferences of sports psychiatrists. *Physician Sport Med.* 2016 Oct 2 [cited 2018 Jul 11];44 (4):397–402. Available from: www.tandfonline.com/doi/full/10.1080/00913847.2016.1216719

13. Malcolm D. Confidentiality in sports medicine. *Clin Sports Med.* 2016;35 (2):205–15.

14. Thomas SA, Merkouris SS, Radermacher HL, Dowling NA, Misso ML, Anderson CJ, et al. Australian guideline for treatment of problem gambling: An abridged outline. *Med J Aust.* 2011 Dec 12;195 (11):664–5.

Cricket: Mental Health Emergencies

Hassan Mahmood and Phil Hopley

Athlete expert advisor: Patrick Foster

Several international cricketers have publicly disclosed their mental health issues in recent years. They have described long days in the field, arduous touring schedules in foreign countries and their experiences of mental health symptoms and disorders. Former professional cricketer Patrick Foster struggled with the boredom of touring and the restrictions that made it hard to find things to stimulate or entertain himself and later found the transition from playing sport and into the real world a huge challenge.

Some media reports have linked poor mental health specifically with cricket and suggested suicide rates are higher compared to other sports. This and other factors have contributed to the development of psychological services within cricket alongside media interest such as a TV series (*Mind Games*) and a short film (*The Edge*), both broadcast in 2019. Playing test cricket requires powers of concentration and mental strength to succeed at the highest level and sports psychologists are already well established in the support teams of major test-playing nations. However, when touring cricketers experience acute mental illness this can present with additional diagnostic and management challenges for the team's MDT staff.

Background

BK is a 25-year-old professional male cricketer who plays for an international team. He has been in the squad for the majority of the last four seasons. Twelve months ago he sustained a right hand injury while fielding in the slips, which meant he was out of action for six months. After making a good recovery, he regained his place in the squad. Two weeks ago during an overseas tour, he was hit in the same area while batting in the nets but was expected to be fit to play again in two to three weeks' time.

Over the last four days his team-mates had become increasingly concerned about his interactions with them in the team environment and the team captain had spoken to the coach to express these concerns. The hotel staff had made a complaint about his over-familiarity. The physiotherapist was worried that he might have taken illicit substances and separately raised concerns with team management. He had been inconsistent with engagement in rehabilitative treatment for his injury.

The team doctor spoke to B and suspected that he was currently experiencing symptoms of mental illness. She had not seen anything like this before and had little training or experience in mental health. She had spoken to a friend, a sports psychiatrist with experience of treating elite athletes, and unless B could be persuaded to see a psychiatrist she saw no other option but to send him home for a full assessment. The team coach was becoming angry with B around the team, wanted him to go home immediately and felt this was an unwelcome distraction for everyone before an important upcoming test match. B therefore agreed to the team doctor referring him to the sports psychiatrist for an online video consultation. The team doctor appreciated this was far from ideal, but with limited resources or other options available, hoped this might work. Thankfully, B, although reluctant, agreed to this. A copy of the sports psychiatrist's consultation is outlined below.

Presenting Complaint

'Mate it's nothing really; my team-mates think I'm getting carried away a bit.'

History of Presenting Complaint

B presented with a four-day history of sleeping for three to four hours per night, which is much less than his usual eight hours or more per night. He denied fatigue and felt full of energy. This had been building up a few weeks before his right hand was re-injured. He was frustrated that he could not play in the next match but said he was 'enjoying the touring experience'.

'I feel great, I don't need to sleep that much, it's great fun going out at night and waking up pretty early, I feel better than ever.'

B believed that he should already have returned to play as it is 'only a soft tissue injury'. He was insistent that he should be deemed fit for the final test match starting in two days. The medical team were equally adamant that he could not play based on their assessment and his attempted rehabilitation.

At times, B believed the team could not cope without him although he acknowledged that his replacement was an experienced test batsman in good form and 'more importantly a great guy who I love'.

Due to B becoming impatient about missing a team meeting (from which he had already been excused), he was in too much of a rush to be able to provide more information. He became irritated by being questioned and asked if the consultation could finish as soon as possible. On brief direct questioning there were no symptoms of depression or anxiety following his injury. He denied experiencing hallucinations.

Past Psychiatric History

He had no past psychiatric history and specifically no previous history of mood disorder episodes or substance misuse problems.

Family History

His paternal uncle had been given a diagnosis of bipolar affective disorder and admitted to a psychiatric hospital on multiple occasions for treatment of both manic and depressive episodes. He has two sisters with no reported mental health problems. His mother was diagnosed with cancer two years ago and had made a full recovery.

Past Medical History

Twelve months ago, he sustained a dorsal fracture-dislocation of the proximal interphalangeal joint in the third finger of his right hand while fielding in the slips. This required surgery (reduction and insertion of a Kirschner wire) followed by extensive physiotherapy, which meant he was out of action for six months. After making a good recovery, he regained his place in the team.

Two years ago, he had back spasms in the middle of a test match and therefore spent the majority of the next two games off the field.

There was no history of concussions.

He had a full range of blood tests during a recent annual medical which were all within normal range and included full blood count, urea and electrolytes, liver function tests (LFT), bone profile and TFTs.

A recent mandatory random UDS before the tour was clear.

Medication History

B was taking paracetamol 1g four times a day although he had forgotten to take this on occasions.

He had no known drug allergies.

Alcohol and Drug History

He had never used illicit substances and was a non-smoker. He normally did not consume alcohol, but had been consuming vodka during his visits to nightclubs for each of the last three nights, and had been unable to recall how much he had consumed. He had not experienced any alcohol withdrawal symptoms and denied ever having a hangover.

Personal History

There were no reported complications during the pregnancy that resulted in his birth. He was born through normal delivery at term and achieved normal developmental milestones. He was hyperactive as a child, which was normalised by family and teachers due to his cricketing talents. He did not obtain any formal educational qualifications at school. He was popular at school and spent most of his spare time playing cricket. His parents were supportive of his sporting pursuits.

B had been a gifted cricketer since he started playing the sport aged eight years and excelled in school teams. He had always been a top order left-handed batsman and reliable slip fielder. He played adult club cricket from age 14 as well as in national age-group teams. He was signed for the senior regional team when he was 18. His ability to consistently score runs and accelerate the scoring rate when required attracted the attention of national selectors at under-19 level. He played regularly for the regional team for the last five years and had an outstanding record with an average of 50 in four-day cricket and 40 (strike rate 90 per 100 balls) in list A domestic 50-over one-day cricket. He played a key role in several overseas test series and one-day international victories in a variety of conditions while becoming a popular member of the team. There have been no off-field issues until now.

He lived with his parents in the town of his birth until he became engaged five years ago and moved to live with his fiancée in their own home in a major city. They married three years ago and have two daughters, aged one and two. His wife worked part-time as an accountant. They are financially comfortable. His parents and siblings live approximately 150 miles away.

Pre-Morbid Personality

He described himself as always being sociable. He made friends easily and was described by team-mates and others as outgoing and popular. He acknowledged that his mood had increased over the last four days, but not as much as others suggested.

Forensic History

He had no forensic history.

Collateral History

B refused to allow anyone else but the team doctor to be asked about him and his difficulties. A member of hotel staff had informed the team doctor that B had sent inappropriate private messages to her via social media. He had asked other hotel staff in detail about their families and personal interests and had been making those around him feel awkward. He had been seen sneaking out to bars in the evenings. On one occasion, he went to a nightclub and brought a woman back to the hotel where they had unprotected sex. This was despite him being in a stable relationship for the last five years. Team-mates reported that he had been particularly disruptive during team meetings, shouting about how great his team were and how they were going to slaughter the opposition. His coach had become annoyed at him for disrupting net practice by trying to bowl spin when the batsmen on the team are facing 'proper' bowlers in practice. While walking in the hotel lobby, a team-mate saw him drop gambling slips although he was not known to frequent betting shops or casinos or known to have any interest in gambling. The coach had said 'he can't stay on tour' and had put pressure on the team doctor to 'get him home and sort him out'.

Mental State Examination

B was well-kempt and of average build. He was wearing a tight pink shirt, team-issued tracksuit bottoms and an unbranded bright yellow cap. He was carrying a cricket bat around with him and was playing 'air shots' prior to the assessment starting. He had some pressure of speech and was hard to interrupt frequently throughout the video consultation, although seemed to engage better with direct questioning. He was over-familiar in the initial stages, attempted jokes and asked several times about the duration of the call. B was avoidant in discussing the reasons for the consultation and repeatedly asked the meaning behind questions being posed to him. He was restless throughout the assessment, which meant that his face went off the screen regularly. He left the consultation on two occasions for a drink of water but was coaxed back by the team doctor. He vented his frustrations about his hand injury incongruently and insisted he could play the next test match despite his injury, even though his medical team had deemed him unfit to play. His mood was objectively elated and this persisted for the duration of the consultation. He had no thoughts or plans of deliberate self-harm (DSH) or suicide. He had no thoughts or plans of harming others. He did not present with grandiose delusions, persecutory delusions, thought interference symptoms or passivity phenomena. He was not responding to unseen stimuli. His insight into his behaviour when among others in the team environment, alcohol consumption and the severity of his injury were all impaired. He acknowledged that his mood had increased a little but did not see this as a problem. He did not have any concerns about his alcohol consumption although agreed it was uncharacteristic and he believed he was fit to play despite his injury.

Risk Assessment

Self: He had no thoughts or plans of DSH or suicide and there was no history of DSH or suicide attempts. His sleep had been very poor and he had been consuming alcohol in quantities that he cannot recall. He had been gambling and at risk of significant overspending.

Others: He had no thoughts or plans of harming others and there was no forensic history. There was a potential risk from others resulting from his over-familiarity. This might make him vulnerable to exploitation. In addition, he was known to have had unprotected sexual intercourse likely related to alcohol intoxication and disinhibition.

Protective factors: there was some motivation to engage in professional support and he had agreed to a consultation. However, his insight into his mental state disturbance was incomplete and this may compromise his ability to agree to an appropriate treatment plan.

Formulation

B presented as a 25-year-old male professional international cricketer who played test and one-day internationals for his country. He had possessed elevated mood for the past four days, increased energy, pressure of speech, decreased need for sleep, distractibility with an effect on both social and occupational functioning. This had occurred following a recent re-injury to his right hand. His presentation strongly suggested a hypomanic episode. More prolonged symptoms (seven days or more), higher severity symptoms (e.g. grandiose delusions or other psychotic symptoms) and greater functional impairment (e.g. a high level of risk requiring hospitalisation) would have indicated a manic rather than a hypomanic episode. While the severity of his symptoms had been close to the threshold for diagnosing the latter, the duration was deemed too short.

A paternal uncle had a diagnosis of bipolar affective disorder, pointing to a genetic predisposition to this disorder. Perpetuating factors included frustration about not being able to play as advised by the team doctor and being within a different social environment. Sleep deprivation may also have been contributing towards further elevation of mood and uncharacteristic use of alcohol, leading to further disinhibition and 'risky' behaviours. Illicit substances (e.g. amphetamines, cocaine and other psycho-stimulants) can precipitate a similar clinic picture or contribute to the deterioration of an emerging hypomanic or manic episode and where possible should always be excluded. He denied any such use and corroborative histories from his team were consistent with this; nonetheless it would be important to screen for potential substance use.

B was isolated from family support and although motivated to engage in professional support this was primarily the result of encouragement from others. He did not fully acknowledge the nature or extent of the recent disturbance in his mood.

Plan

- Medication was very likely to be required and would be offered. During acute hypomania/mania, antipsychotics medications can have a rapid anti-manic effect and

can be augmented with benzodiazepines. He was offered olanzapine 10mg to be repeated daily and diazepam 2mg to be repeated as required
- There should be a sensitive exploration into whether recreational substances have contributed to his symptoms. Stimulant use can be associated with examination signs such as dilated pupils and tics. A urine sample is informative if the result is positive but a negative sample does not always exclude use
- Simple psychological interventions can be helpful to de-escalate behavioural disturbance. Multiple interactions with others can be confusing and even cause escalation but simple reassurance and orientation from one clinician or staff member can be calming and help engage him verbally. Active listening in a quiet and calm space is more likely to establish collaboration
- During recovery, as his mood returns to normal, he would benefit from advice on both alcohol and gambling and if necessary specific interventions to address these areas
- Debriefing with a qualified mental health clinician as his condition improves would help him to develop prevention strategies for future episodes
- His recent presentation was not compatible with playing elite-level sport and team management had indicated that he would not be taking any further part on the current tour. He would benefit from being around his familiar home environment and therefore closer to greater MDT professional support
- He would be chaperoned home in order to receive a more formal and thorough assessment. As he is well known to the public, the national cricket board had commissioned a private aeroplane for him to return home. This was to maintain his confidentiality and reduce the risk of further overspending and alcohol consumption
- The team doctor had been asked to liaise with B's family, who will meet him at the airport and accompany him back to his home
- The team doctor and the sports psychiatrist arranged for him to have a formal psychiatric evaluation within 48 hours of arriving home

Questions

Q 1 Which of the following statements are correct?
   A. Assessment of elite athletes experiencing a mental health emergency should follow an approach that is different to other mental health assessments
   B. Values that guide an appropriate emergency response include avoiding physical and emotional harm, using person-centred approaches with shared responsibility, respect and use of an individual's strengths and natural support networks and establishing safety
   C. There is available data on the prevalence of bipolar and psychotic disorders in elite athletes
   D. Mental health emergency plans should be consistent with other emergencies in sport
   E. In the acute management of suicide or self-harm risk in an athlete, it is important to ensure the immediate safety of the athlete only

Q 2 B is initially treated with an antipsychotic medication, but with limited anti-manic effect. Treatment with a second antipsychotic medication up to British National Formulary maximum dose causes no side effects. However, despite an improvement in his mental state, he continues to present with some residual symptoms of hypomania. What would be the appropriate additional treatment at this stage?

A. Antidepressant medication

B. CBT

C. Inpatient admission

D. Disulfiram

E. Mood stabilising medication

Q 3   B has appropriate treatment for his episode of hypomania. Six months later, he presents with a three-week history of persistent low mood for no obvious reason with anhedonia, poor sleep, lack of energy, poor concentration, low self-esteem, reduced appetite, weight loss and excessive feelings of guilt. There are no hallucinations or delusions. He has no suicidal thoughts. What is the diagnosis?

A. Schizophrenia

B. Bipolar affective disorder, current episode severe depression with psychotic symptoms

C. Bipolar affective disorder, current episode severe depression without psychotic symptoms

D. Mild depressive episode

E. Mania without psychotic symptoms

Q 4   Which of the following statements are correct regarding bipolar affective disorder?

A. At least 90% of patients with mania experience further episodes of major mood disturbance

B. The interval between episodes becomes progressively longer with both age and the number of episodes

C. Nearly all patients with bipolar affective disorder recover from acute episodes and the long-term prognosis is good

D. Mortality is significantly decreased in patients with bipolar affective disorders

E. All of the above statements are correct

Q 5   B states that he is due to play 20- and 50-over and four-day Championship cricket for an English county in the summer. Support for cricketers regarding mental health will be available if needed during his stint as an overseas player in county cricket. True or False?

Answers

Q 1)   B and D

Like any other assessment in medicine, an assessment of elite athletes experiencing a mental health emergency should follow a structured approach (1,2,3,4) to ensure important elements of the presentation are not missed and that there is some degree of uniformity between professionals. This commences with a thorough history and where possible in a sporting environment should include a collateral history from team-mates, other members of team staff and family.

Values that guide an appropriate emergency response are important. These include avoiding physical and emotional harm, using person-centred approaches with shared responsibility, respect and use of an individual's strengths and natural support networks, establishing safety, and adhering to principles of hope, recovery and resilience as set out in a recent narrative review of the topic (1).

Core parts of a mental health emergency management plan include identifying situations, symptoms or behaviours that are considered mental health emergencies. Developing written procedures for management of various mental health emergencies should be a priority for sporting administrations. In B's case, the team doctor was fortunate to know a sports psychiatrist, but the team doctor could put together these procedures with the support of a psychiatrist in B's home country in planning for the future. In a pre-emptive measure, it would be helpful for a team doctor, sports psychiatrist, psychology services, players, masseurs, physiotherapists, coaches, management and any others travelling with the team to work together to identify responsibilities and roles in identifying mental health symptoms and their subsequent management. This is something that a sports psychiatrist should have expertise in co-ordinating.

There is no available data on the prevalence of bipolar and psychotic disorders in elite athletes (1,5,6,7,8). However, bipolar affective disorder and the spectrum of psychotic disorders are among the most common mental health disorders seen within the general population and the typical age of onset coincides with peak performance age of elite athletes (9). This increases the importance of all in the elite sporting environment being made aware of the symptoms of bipolar and psychotic disorders. They have a significant impact on quality of life and functioning, which, in the context of elite sport, includes a negative impact on sporting performance (8). A narrative review of bipolar disorder in elite athletes describes how history, clinical features and physical examination can be used to distinguish between primary bipolar and psychotic disorders and those secondary to substance misuse in sport (8). This is a key part of any related presenting complaint and will guide management.

Q 2) E

B has been treated in accordance with UK national guidelines (10). If expected outcomes have not occurred an important first step is to check adherence with medication. As the second antipsychotic was not sufficiently effective at the maximum licensed dose, lithium should be considered. Lithium stabilises mood during the acute phases of the illness, prevents relapse in both mania and depression, and reduces the risk of suicide (11). Investigations are required before commencing treatment and regular blood monitoring is needed once treatment is established (12). Common side effects include fine tremor, gastrointestinal disturbances (e.g. nausea, diarrhoea), polyuria, metallic taste, polydipsia and weight gain. Other adverse effects to look out for include: changes in thyroid function, oedema, exacerbations of skin disorders (e.g. psoriasis, acne) and electrocardiogram (ECG) changes.

For patients taking lithium, treatment guidelines suggest; 'ensure they maintain their fluid intake, particularly after sweating (e.g. after exercise, in hot climates or if they have a fever), if they are immobile for long periods or if they develop an infection' (10). In addition, some evidence suggests that sweating reduces lithium levels (13). B mainly plays his cricket in warm climates. It will be important for him to be briefed on self-management to prevent dehydration during extensive periods in the field (minimising the risk of lithium toxicity) and the need for close monitoring when there is heavy sweating (to prevent lithium levels dropping below the therapeutic threshold). Vigilance and increased monitoring are needed when people become physically unwell or medications are added that might interfere with renal clearance, e.g. non-steroidal anti-inflammatory drugs (11).

Valproate is another mood-stabilising medication that can be considered. When starting valproate, weight and BMI should be measured alongside a FBC and LFTs. These should be re-checked after six months and repeated on an annual basis once medication is stabilised. If valproate were commenced, he would need to be advised about recognising signs and symptoms of blood and liver disorders (including obvious signs as bruising or jaundice and those that may be less obvious such as general fatigue and sweating) and to seek immediate medical attention if any develop (11). Medication should be stopped immediately if there are abnormal LFT or blood abnormalities (11). Valproate is not prescribed to women of childbearing potential as there is a risk of foetal malformations and adverse neuro-developmental outcomes after any exposure in pregnancy.

Managing Lithium Toxicity

An example guideline (www.iow.nhs.uk/Pharmacy/Documents/Lithium%20prescribing% 20guidelines%202014.pdf) states:

- Patients are at particular risk from this when there are changes to sodium levels, e.g. low-sodium diets, dehydration, drug interactions and some physical illnesses (e.g. Addison's disease)
- Toxic effects typically occur at levels >1.5 mmol/l and usually include: Gastrointestinal effects, increasing anorexia, nausea and diarrhoea
- Central nervous system effects: muscle weakness, drowsiness, ataxia, coarse tremor and muscle twitching
- Above 2 mmol/l, increased disorientation and seizures usually occur, which can progress to coma and ultimately death
- If a patient exhibits signs of lithium toxicity:
  1) Stop lithium immediately
  2) Check lithium levels and renal function
  3) Refer to hospital if clinical condition warrants
  4) Seek advice from psychiatrist for re-initiation of lithium
- In the presence of more severe symptoms, osmotic or forced alkaline diuresis should be used; above 3 mmol/l; peritoneal or haemodialysis is often used

Q 3) C

This current episode is indicative of a severe depression without psychotic symptoms and it has occurred in the context of bipolar affective disorder (14) as he has had at least one authenticated hypomanic, manic or mixed affective episode in the past.

Treatment of a depressive episode of this kind requires a broad approach and psychological, social and pharmacological interventions should all be considered. CBT, IPT and family interventions can all be used but their evidence is largely extrapolated from their use in unipolar depression (10,15). No sports-specific psychological interventions have been formally evaluated (8).

Pharmacological management of his depressive episode as per NICE guidelines (10) would include consideration of fluoxetine (a SSRI) combined with olanzapine (an antipsychotic) or the addition of quetiapine (an antipsychotic) depending on the preference of the individual and previous response to treatment. Lurasidone can also be considered (11).

It is important to consider issues especially important to athletes when prescribing psychiatric medications. These include side effects, safety concerns and anti-doping policies. Sports psychiatrists should be mindful of which type of athlete they are providing care for and player expectations as a result – this can often guide management more so than in the general population. Sports-specific treatments have not been investigated but expert opinion in sports psychiatry has recommended quetiapine, lurasidone and lamotrigine as suitable treatments in bipolar depression (8). Lamotrigine and lurasidone are less sedating and have fewer metabolic and cardiac concerns. Invited physician members of the ISSP completed an anonymous web-based survey on psychiatric medication prescribing preferences in working with athletes with a variety of mental health conditions. Lamotrigine was the first choice for bipolar spectrum disorders and prescribing preferences for athletes were different to prescribing trends seen in the general population, which matched the assumption that different factors are considered when prescribing for athletes (8).

As with management of any acutely unwell patient, a comprehensive risk assessment should be completed and documented. Psychiatrists should take into account the toxicity of psychotropic medications in overdose when prescribing and adjust treatment plans to contribute to risk minimisation. While psychotropic drugs have an established efficacy in treating psychiatric conditions, there is evidence of a link between increased prescribing rates and increased use in intentional drug overdose (16).

There are some similarities and differences between NICE guidelines and British Association of Pharmacology (BAP) guidelines for long-term treatment. Both recommend lithium as first-line treatment but NICE recommends considering adding valproate if lithium is ineffective while BAP is more specific and recommends additional treatment with lamotrigine, quetiapine or lurasidone if depression is predominant or valproate or dopamine antagonist/partial agonist if mania is predominant. If lithium is poorly tolerated or unsuitable, valproate, olanzapine, quetiapine or other dopamine antagonists/partial agonists can all be considered for long-term prophylaxis (10,11).

Psycho-education (the process of providing education and information to those seeking or receiving mental health services) is an important intervention in any sphere of mental health and can be especially useful in the long-term management of bipolar disorder (10,15,17). This includes informing him and close family/carers about the long-term relapsing and remitting nature of the condition and self-management strategies to address factors that can destabilise the illness.

Q 4) A

The onset of bipolar disorder tends to be present within the first two to three decades of life. It is important to be mindful of transcultural factors when considering mood disorders as patients from minority groups are more likely to present with a first episode of mania and prominent psychotic features compared to a white European population (18). Other general information summarised below can assist a clinician in discussing the future prognosis with patients (12):

- The age of onset of bipolar disorder is typically about 21 years in hospital studies, but earlier (about 18 years) in community surveys. Late-onset bipolar disorder is rare and should prompt a careful search for possible organic brain disease
- Bipolar disorder usually presents initially with depression with the first manic episode manifesting on average five years later
- Around 90% of patients with mania experience further mood episodes
- The interval between episodes becomes progressively shorter with both age and the number of episodes
- While many patients have a good recovery from acute episodes, the long-term prognosis is less good and residual symptoms are common

Mortality is significantly increased in patients with bipolar disorders. Over a 40-year follow up, 8% of men and 5% of women who had been hospitalised for a bipolar illness died by suicide (19). General medical conditions such as cardiovascular disease and the secondary consequences of co-morbid substance misuse, including smoking, also contribute to the high mortality observed. A study of approximately 22,000 Danish patients with bipolar disorder found a reduction in life expectancy of approximately 13 years in men and 9 years in women. About two-thirds of this reduction was accounted for by natural causes, with the remainder being due to suicide and accidents (20). The long-term management of bipolar disorder needs to consider not only the relatively high suicide burden but also the cardio-vascular risk and appropriate lifestyle interventions.

Q 5) True

Cricketers sharing their experiences of mental illness has directly contributed to the development of programmes to address mental health concerns in this sport.

The Players Cricket Association (PCA) in England provides many aspects of education and support for physical and mental wellbeing. PCA and Mind (a leading mental health charity) deliver workshops on mental wellbeing to professional cricket academies in England and Wales. Since 2018, they have been delivering educational sessions on understanding and supporting an individual's mental health (www.thepca.co.uk/press-release/pca-personal-development-programme/). PCA mental health ambassadors, a PCA 'stress-free' app and signposting for support with emotional management and mental health concerns and conditions are also all available. 'Mind Fit' sessions have also been introduced and focus on supporting players' mental wellbeing. These sessions have five components:

1. What is mental health?
2. Why is it important to talk about mental health?
3. When to seek support: early warning signs
4. How to manage stress and support wellbeing
5. Where to get support

Other countries have also been active in this area and the Australian Cricket Association (ACA) jointly runs 'The Professional Development Program' with Cricket Australia (www.auscricket.com.au/game-plan/pd-program). It is available to current players, those who have recently retired and some past players (on a case-by-case basis). The programme includes provision for wellbeing and health services (including access to counselling); support with career transition; grants and other support for further education and a player hardship fund. The ACA and Cricket Australia provide confidential counselling to members and their families through partnership with Relationships Australia. A similar programme exists in the New Zealand Cricket Players Association. Less is known about mental health support available in other major cricketing nations such as Pakistan, India, Sri Lanka and Bangladesh.

> ### Summary of the Chapter and the Topics Covered
>
> * Managing mental health illness emergencies in elite athletes
> * Treatment of hypomania
> * Diagnosing bipolar affective disorder
> * Long-term outcomes of people with bipolar affective disorders
> * Mental health support availability for professional cricketers around the world

References

1. Currie A, McDuff D, Johnston A, Hopley P, Hitchcock ME, Reardon CL, et al. Management of mental health emergencies in elite athletes: A narrative review. *Br J Sports Med*. 2019 [cited 2019 May 17]; bjsports-2019-100691. Available from: http://bjsm.bmj.com/lookup/doi/10.1136/bjsports-2019-100691

2. Currie A, Johnston A. Psychiatric disorders: The psychiatrist's contribution to sport. *Int Rev Psychiatry*. 2016 [cited 2016 Dec 7];28(6):587–94. Available from: www.tandfonline.com/doi/full/10.1080/09540261.2016.1197188

3. Kamm RL. Interviewing principles for the psychiatrically aware sports medicine physician. *Clin Sports Med*. 2005 [cited 2016 Nov 21];24(4):745–69. Available from: http://linkinghub.elsevier.com/retrieve/pii/S0278591905000463

4. Silverman JJ, Galanter M, Jackson-Triche M, Jacobs DG, Lomax JW, Riba MB, et al. The American Psychiatric Association practice guidelines for the psychiatric evaluation of adults. *Am J Psychiatry*. 2015 [cited 2018 Dec 10];172(8):798–802. Available from: www.ncbi.nlm.nih.gov/pubmed/26234607

5. Reardon CL. Psychiatric comorbidities in sports. *Neurol Clin*. 2017 [cited 2018 Apr 20];35(3):537–46. Available from: www.ncbi.nlm.nih.gov/pubmed/28673414

6. Reardon CL, Factor RM. Sport psychiatry: A systematic review of diagnosis and medical treatment of mental illness in athletes. *Sport Med*. 2010;40(11):961–80. Available from: http://ovidsp.ovid.com/ovidweb.cgi?T=JS&PAGE=reference&D=med5&NEWS=N&AN=20942511%5Cnhttp://link.springer.com/10.2165/11536580-000000000-00000

7. Rice SM, Purcell R, De Silva S, Mawren D, McGorry PD, Parker AG. The mental health of elite athletes: A narrative systematic review. *Sport Med*. 2016;46(9):1333–53. Available from: http://dx.doi.org/10.1007/s40279-016-0492-2

8. Currie A, Gorczynski P, Rice SM, Purcell R, McAllister-Williams RH, Hitchcock ME, et al. Bipolar and psychotic disorders in elite athletes: A narrative review. *Br J Sports Med*. 2019 [cited 2019 May 17];bjsports-2019-100685. Available from: http://bjsm.bmj.com/lookup/doi/10.1136/bjsports-2019-100685

9. Moesch K, Kenttä G, Kleinert J, Quignon-Fleuret C, Cecil S, Bertollo M. FEPSAC position statement: Mental health disorders in elite athletes and models of service provision. *Psychol Sport Exerc*. 2018;38:61–71. Available from: www.sciencedirect.com/science/article/pii/S1469029218300153

10. National Institute for Health and Care Excellence. *Bipolar Disorder (update): the assessment and management of bipolar disorder in adults, children and young people in primary and secondary care*. 2014.

11. Goodwin GM, Haddad PM, Ferrier IN, Aronson JK, Barnes TRH, Cipriani A, et al. Evidence-based guidelines for treating

bipolar disorder: Revised third edition recommendations from the British Association for Psychopharmacology. *J Psychopharmacol.* 2016;30(6):495–553.

12. Harrison P, Cowen P, Burns T, Fazel M. Bipolar disorder. In: Harrison P, Cowen P, Burns T, Fazel M, eds. *Shorter Oxford Textbook of Psychiatry.* 7th edition. Oxford University Press; 2017 [cited 2019 Dec 6]. p. 233–52. Available from: www .oxfordmedicine.com/view/10.1093/med/9 780198747437.001.0001/med-9780198747 437-chapter-10

13. Reardon CL. The sports psychiatrist and psychiatric medication. *Int Rev Psychiatry.* 2016 [cited 2016 Dec 7];28(6):606–13. Available from: www.tandfonline.com/doi/ full/10.1080/09540261.2016.1190691

14. World Health Organization. *International Statistical Classification of Diseases and Related Health Problems – 10th Revision.* World Health Organization. 2011.

15. Hirschfield RMA, Bowden CL, Gitlin MJ, Keck PE, Suppes T, Thase ME, et al. *Treatment of Patients with Bipolar Disorder.* 2nd edition. (Practice Guideline) American Psychological Association. 2010; (December): p. 1–82.

16. Corcoran P, Heavey B, Griffin E, Perry IJ, Arensman E. Psychotropic medication involved in intentional drug overdose: Implications for treatment. *Neuropsychiatry (London).* 2013;3(3):285–93.

17. Colom F, Vieta E, Reinares M, Martínez-Arán A, Torrent C, Goikolea JM, et al. Psychoeducation efficacy in bipolar disorders: Beyond compliance enhancement. *J Clin Psychiatry.* 2003 [cited 2019 Jan 31];64(9):1101–5. Available from: www.ncbi.nlm.nih.gov/p ubmed/14628987

18. Kennedy N, Boydell J, Van Os J, Murray RM. Ethnic differences in first clinical presentation of bipolar disorder: Results from an epidemiological study. *J Affect Disord.* 2004;83(2–3):161–8.

19. Nordentoft M, Mortensen PB, Pedersen CB. Absolute risk of suicide after first hospital contact in mental disorder. *Arch Gen Psychiatry.* 2011;68 (10):1058–64.

20. Kessing LV, Vradi E, McIntyre RS, Andersen PK. Causes of decreased life expectancy over the life span in bipolar disorder. *J Affect Disord.* 2015 15;180:142–7.

Cycling: Attention Deficit Hyperactivity Disorder and Anti-Doping

James Dove

Athlete expert advisor: Luke Rowe

Attention deficit hyperactivity disorder (ADHD) carries a high personal, social and economic burden. Those with the disorder have a high incidence of co-morbid depression and anxiety as well as substance misuse disorders. There is particular sensitivity around the diagnosis in elite sport given that the first-line pharmacological therapy for treatment of ADHD remains stimulant medications, which are prohibited substances requiring a therapeutic use exemption (TUE). Any psychiatric assessment should consider the disorder in adults and sports psychiatrists in particular have a responsibility to assess, diagnose, treat and educate athletes and teams about the need for treatment and the legislation governing stimulant use in elite sport.

Background

SG is a 25-year-old professional track cyclist whose new team coach of six months had become increasingly concerned by S's erratic behaviour and loss of form during the off-season. The coach felt that he had explored all other avenues of what could be preventing S from performing at his best.

From a young age, S was introduced to cycling as a way to channel his high energy levels. His mother would describe him as often, 'bouncing off the walls'. Despite being a highly talented cyclist, he would often struggle with basic instructions given by coaching teams. During his schooling years he was diagnosed with dyslexia and required support from an educational psychologist.

S was worried that his coach wanted to drop him from the new team and reluctantly agreed to attend an outpatient consultation with a recommended sports psychiatrist. A copy of the subsequent psychiatric assessment has been outlined below.

Presenting Complaint

'I'm really anxious that my new team are going to drop me, I just can't seem to focus.'

History of Presenting Complaint

S presented to the clinic in a state of considerable distress, visibly sweating. He stated that he had been with his new cycling team for six months and had struggled to focus at training sessions, often getting distracted and constantly losing his new kit. Also, S was very concerned about a recent loss of form as well as having received a driving ban for repeat speeding offences.

S was worried that this assessment was part of his team management's plan to gather evidence so that they could drop him from the cycling squad. When asked about symptoms of inattention and hyperactivity he stated that he struggled to complete tasks and was finding it hard to understand the new tasks related to his new training regime. He reported that he struggled to follow instructions of more than two stages and would like his new coach to break down stages for him.

He also reported multiple mistakes in planning and particular problems related to remembering to do day-to-day tasks. S stated, 'everyone always says that I make silly mistakes, I just can't seem to help it'. S disclosed that he was just starting to familiarise himself with the coach's post-lap 'cue card' instruction system to help him remember next cycling stages. Recently, S had set up regular alarms and reminders on his phone to ensure that he turned up to training sessions on time and brought the appropriate training kit and bike gear.

On reflection, S missed his old coach who had managed him since he was 13 years old. He felt he had been able to understand him better and he had always given him positive encouragement. He believed that moving to this new team had destabilised him and that he was unsure as to what was now expected of him. S admitted that his cigarette smoking habit had re-surfaced and this disappointed him.

Past Psychiatric History

S was referred to an educational psychologist as a teenager (aged 15) because of poor school performance and truanting. He was diagnosed with dyslexia and offered extra educational support.

Family History

Nothing was known: S believed his father had had a psychiatric assessment but he did not know the outcome of this.

Past Medical History

S has had rib fractures and surgery for a clavicular fracture following cycling accidents.
There was no history of acute head injuries or concussion.

Medication

No regular medication or psychotropic medication in the past.
No known drug allergies.

Social History

S was single and lived with his mother in the North of England. However, he was often abroad competing and training at various cycling events. His parents separated when he was nine years old following his father's arrest for dealing class A drugs. His father was subsequently imprisoned. His mother was employed as a nursery nurse and his father was now out of prison but had not returned to work. S had very limited contact with his estranged father.

S had always avoided drugs and alcohol since his father's arrest and imprisonment, viewing them as 'unnecessary evils'. He had always had too much energy anyway and feared the potential effect they would have on him. He admitted to very occasionally smoking cigarettes while feeling anxious but managed to limit this to once a week during the off-season period.

Personal History

S denied experiencing any complications at birth and had achieved all his normal developmental milestones without any delay. S reported that he never enjoyed school. He found the transition from primary to secondary education particularly difficult as this also occurred around the time of his father's trouble with the police and when his parents had separated. He began truanting at the age of 11 but did not receive his dyslexia diagnosis until he was aged 15. His father was a keen cyclist and S attended a local road cycling club and went to track days with him from a young age.

By the time S was 15 he had dropped out of school to focus on cycling both road and track, ultimately focusing on the individual pursuit with considerable success locally and nationally, narrowly missing Olympic selection at the age of 22. Since then he had struggled to retain his form and had had a number of driving incidents recently leading to him being disqualified from driving a vehicle for the next six months.

Pre-Morbid Personality

S had always been somewhat irritable and suspicious of people, struggling to maintain relationships and sustain long-lasting friendships. He stated that cycling was the only thing he had ever been good at and that this was the entire focus of his life. S reported that he was particularly good at individual pursuit but had always needed a lot of encouragement and support. He was never popular with wider club members as he always needed constant attention to keep him on task. He had never been viewed as much of a team player. S stated that he was not able to reach competition level on long road races as he had always wanted to lead. However, he tended to perform well in time trials and individual pursuit.

Forensic History

S had recently received a six-month driving ban for repeat speeding offences.

S was well known to the police locally in childhood for minor infractions and behavioural concerns but had never been charged with any offences.

Collateral History

S's mother expressed great concerns about her son. She was relieved when he had signed a professional contract but was of the view that he had gone downhill since failing selection for the Olympic team. She felt the fact that he was not diagnosed with reading difficulties (dyslexia) until his teenage years had a big impact on his confidence and prospects as an adult.

She reported that even before his father left he was always 'a handful and bouncing off the walls' both at home and school – she would regularly get calls from school about his disruptive behaviour – both truanting away from lessons and unruly behaviour while in the classroom. She stated that she could not manage him at home and if it had not been for the cycling club holding his attention she was unsure she could have raised him on her own.

During his childhood he could never stay sitting down for a meal or long enough to watch a film. She expressed feeling guilty about being too busy at the time and not getting the professional help that she felt he needed. She prayed that he would settle given his recent cycling successes but was now more concerned about him. She believed that he had become less energetic than he was in childhood and appeared more distracted, less able to focus on tasks or to get anything done, including his beloved cycling.

Mental State Examination

S presented as a young Caucasian male. He was tall and slim, of athletic build and well-kempt. S was wearing a tracksuit and trainers. He appeared upset, agitated and struggled to keep still in his seat. S was visibly sweating. He tapped his fingers on the desk as he spoke and was irritable and somewhat demanding in demeanour. He made only fleeting eye contact. Speech was fast but low volume and mumbled and he interrupted the interviewer frequently. At times S became a little incoherent because of levels of anxiety and emotion. He stated he had felt low in mood for some months and had been struggling to see any positives in life. He reported low energy levels for the same time period and feeling on edge for no apparent reason. S stated that his sleep had been disturbed for some weeks now (difficulty initiating sleep) and that he had little or no appetite and was forcing himself to eat so that he could train. S expressed thoughts of guilt and worthlessness about recent events. He admitted to recent fleeting suicidal thoughts but without plans. He acknowledged his restlessness at the interview but said he is not normally a 'fidgety' person and had felt particularly anxious because of the assessment. There was no evidence of thought disorder or psychotic symptoms. Cognition was not formally tested but he reported concerns about short-term memory relating to his inability to remember basic instructions and complete tasks.

S had some insight in that he recognised that something was not right with his high level of agitation, restlessness and inability to concentrate and remember things. He was very concerned about any mental health diagnosis and stated his reluctance to take any medication that might impact on training or stop him from competing at the highest level.

Risk Assessment

Self: S stated that he had never self-harmed but reported that he felt very anxious and in this current state he did not know what to do or how to contain himself. He stated that he had recently thought about suicide briefly for the first time in his life but denied making any plans to end his life. He was focused on returning to cycling and regaining form as the only positive thing in his life.

Others: No thoughts of harm to others. His recent vehicle driving had been dangerous and unrestrained with recent, inappropriate risk-taking at times punished with repeated speeding offences. This was currently managed by an external control (his driving ban).

Protective factors: S stated that he could never end his life as he could not put his mother through such grief.

Investigations
- Normal blood tests including LFT and TFTs
- ECG showed a tachycardia of 104 bpm but he was noted to be extremely agitated during the procedure. His resting heart rate is known to be in the low 40s. Otherwise a normal ECG was seen
- UDS was negative for illicit substances

Case Formulation
S presented as a 25-year-old single professional cyclist living with his mother. He demonstrated symptoms suggestive of anxiety, possibly in context of an acute stress reaction/adjustment reaction related to recent events in both his personal and professional life. This was against a background of a collateral history highly suggestive of ADHD.

He possessed a vulnerable mental state with symptoms suggestive of a co-morbid mixed anxious/depressed mental state with notable irritability. In the context of possible loss of professional occupation, strong athletic identity and impulsivity/risk-taking behaviours his potential suicide risk should be taken seriously.

Questions
Q 1 Based on current presentation and historical information does S meet diagnostic criteria for a diagnosis of ADHD in adulthood?
   A. Meets diagnostic criteria in one domain only – inattentive subtype
   B. ADHD cannot be diagnosed because of the presence of co-morbid mood disorder
   C. Meets diagnostic criteria in one domain only – hyperactive subtype
   D. Meets diagnostic criteria in both domains – combined type
   E. ADHD cannot be diagnosed because of high level of functioning (elite athlete)

Q 2 Environmental modifications and behavioural management are recommended in all cases of ADHD. What additional treatment should be offered to S to manage his symptoms of ADHD in adulthood?
   A. Mindfulness meditation
   B. Methylphenidate or lisdexamfetamine
   C. He should not be prescribed stimulant medication because these drugs are performance enhancing and hence prohibited by WADA for use by elite athletes under any circumstances
   D. SSRI
   E. Atomoxetine

Q 3 What does evidence suggest is the most effective treatment combination in the long-term management of symptoms of ADHD in adulthood?
   A. CBT plus pharmacotherapy
   B. Pharmacotherapy alone

C. CBT alone

D. Dialectical behavioural therapy (DBT) plus pharmacotherapy

E. There is no evidence to support psychological interventions in the management of adult ADHD

Q 4   This question addresses ADHD TUE policy and process.

Initial application to UKAD for a TUE in respect of stimulant treatment use in a diagnosis of ADHD requires the following:

A. Two independent medical reports from clinicians specialising in ADHD

B. One medical report from a psychiatrist specialising in ADHD

C. One medical report from any clinician (psychiatrist, paediatrician or other expert) specialising in ADHD

D. Two independent medical reports from any clinicians (psychiatrist, paediatrician or other expert) specialising in ADHD

E. One medical report from a psychiatrist specialising in ADHD and who is also a member of the UKAD Register of Psychiatrists

Q 5   With respect to our current understanding of the prevalence of ADHD in elite sport, which of the following statements is true?

A. There is good data across all sports that support a higher prevalence than in the general population

B. In a few sports the prevalence rate of ADHD has been accurately established

C. TUE application rates for stimulant medication are an accurate measure of ADHD prevalence

D. Children with ADHD are attracted to and benefit from participating in certain sports

E. There is some evidence for an excess of ADHD in all professional/elite sports

Answers

Q 1)   A

Assessment suggested that S currently meets diagnostic criteria for inattentive subtype of ADHD as set out in the DSM-V (1). He had more than five symptoms in the inattentive category currently and has done for the last six months. His symptoms had been persistent since before aged 12 and with significant impact on social, academic and occupational functioning. It would appear that his ADHD may have matured from a mixed type in childhood to a more inattentive type and the collateral history from his mother is especially helpful in evaluating this progression.

It would appear that focused activity (cycling) had managed to hold his attention with considerable success through adolescence and early adulthood. Symptoms appear to break through at times of stress in his life, perhaps related to off-season when he was less occupied and perhaps leading to the risk-taking behaviours such as his recent speeding.

ADHD is a neuro-developmental disorder (NDD) typified by core symptoms of inattention, hyperactivity and impulsivity. In keeping with other NDDs it is a spectrum disorder. In common with all psychiatric disorders, diagnosis requires not only the presence of core symptoms but also demonstration of impact on functioning (1,2). Core symptoms coupled with deficits in executive function, emotional regulation and motivation can lead to the persistence of the disorder into adulthood (3).

ADHD has classically been recognised as a disorder of childhood but more recently it has been identified that a significant cohort of patients will have symptoms which persist into adulthood. In addition, there are some for whom the diagnosis only comes later in life. Estimates for those experiencing persistent symptoms of ADHD into adulthood range from 60 to 75% of those diagnosed in childhood (4,5). There is an estimated prevalence of 2–5% of the population for the disorder in adulthood (6,7). In keeping with the disorder's categorisation as an NDD, diagnosis in adulthood requires symptoms to be present before the age of 12 (1).

The WHO's International Classification of Diseases (ICD-10) defines a similar disorder of 'hyperkinetic disorder (F90)' (2) with somewhat more restrictive diagnostic criteria than DSM-V. Use of DSM-V criteria is recommended by the worldwide authority on doping in sport (WADA) and therefore also the UK agency: UK Anti-Doping (UKAD). It is also the preferred criteria for both the Royal College of Psychiatrists' guidance on adult ADHD assessment (2017) (8) and the recent IOC consensus statement on mental health in elite athletes (9).

As per DSM-V guidelines, a diagnosis of ADHD is based on the symptoms that have occurred over the past six months. Symptoms are required to have been present since before the age of 12, be present in two or more settings, occur with clear evidence of impact on functioning and do not occur exclusively in the context of a psychotic or other mental disorder. Core symptom clusters are as follows (1):

Inattentive type – six (or five for people over 17 years) of the following symptoms occur frequently:

- Does not pay close attention to details or makes careless mistakes in school or job tasks
- Has problems staying focused on tasks or activities, such as during lectures, conversations or long reading
- Does not seem to listen when spoken to (i.e. seems to be elsewhere)
- Does not follow through on instructions and does not complete schoolwork, chores or job duties (may start tasks but quickly loses focus)
- Has problems organising tasks and work (for instance, does not manage time well; has messy, disorganised work; misses deadlines)
- Avoids or dislikes tasks that require sustained mental effort, such as preparing reports and completing forms
- Often loses things needed for tasks or daily life, such as school papers, books, keys, wallet, cell phone and eyeglasses
- Is easily distracted
- Forgets daily tasks, such as doing chores and running errands. Older teens and adults may forget to return phone calls, pay bills and keep appointments

Hyperactive/impulsive type – six (or five for people over 17 years) of the following symptoms occur frequently:

- Fidgets with or taps hands or feet, or squirms in seat
- Not able to stay seated (in classroom, workplace)
- Runs about or climbs where it is inappropriate
- Unable to play or do leisure activities quietly

- Always 'on the go', as if driven by a motor
- Talks too much
- Blurts out an answer before a question has been finished (for instance may finish people's sentences, cannot wait to speak in conversations)
- Has difficulty waiting his or her turn, such as while waiting in line
- Interrupts or intrudes on others (for instance, cuts into conversations, games or activities, or starts using other people's things without permission). Older teens and adults may take over what others are doing

Although severe mental illness is an exclusion criteria for the diagnosis of ADHD (schizophrenia, bipolar disorder and substance misuse disorder) (1), co-morbidity in ADHD should be considered the 'rule not the exception' where chronic mood instability should be considered 'part of the core syndrome of ADHD' (6). It is also recognised that mood instability (mild/moderate symptoms of depression and anxiety) may respond well to the treatment of the core symptoms of ADHD, and should not preclude the use of stimulant medication as first-line treatment (8).

A total of 75% of those with a diagnosis of ADHD in adulthood have at least one co-morbid mental illness with the most common being mood disorders, personality disorders and substance misuse disorders (6).

Q 2)   B

S presented with symptoms of untreated ADHD having been assessed and diagnosed by a psychiatrist. First-line treatment in all cases is environmental modifications. NICE (10) highlights noise reduction and anti-distraction techniques as well as simple strategies to increase focus on task/work. In the presence of 'significant impairment in at least one domain' stimulant medication such as methylphenidate can also be offered. This should be done following a specialist assessment and discussion between psychiatrist and patient on treatment preferences and risk factors (10).

Common side effects of stimulant medication include weight loss, insomnia, abdominal pain, decreased appetite, dry mouth and sexual dysfunction (11). Close monitoring of side effects is necessary in elite athletes, including awareness that stimulants can lead to an ability to tolerate increased core body temperature during exercise and mask signs of thermal stress (12).

Athletes competing in sport are subject to anti-doping responsibilities relating to their medical treatment. The WADA prohibited list, published on an annual basis, sets out the substances and methods which are prohibited in sport. The list is divided into substances and methods which are 'prohibited at all times' and 'prohibited in-competition only' (12). Stimulant medications, including those used to treat ADHD, are prohibited in-competition only (5). Athletes who are prescribed a prohibited medication are required to obtain a TUE.

Atomoxetine (a noradrenaline reuptake inhibitor) is considered second-line pharmacotherapy in adult ADHD for those that do not tolerate stimulant medication (10). It is a permitted medication as is not on the WADA prohibited list (12) and therefore does not require a TUE. However, there is no requirement to trial atomoxetine as a first-line treatment in athletes, prior to the prescription of a stimulant medication (13).

Patients diagnosed with ADHD and prescribed stimulant medication should be aware that ADHD is a Driving and Vehicle Licensing Agency (DVLA) notifiable condition. It is the responsibility of the person diagnosed to inform the DVLA so a decision can be made on the appropriateness of driving depending on symptom burden and treatment plan (14). It has been noted that risk of driving offences is higher in those with ADHD, particularly speeding offences, possibly linked to thrill-seeking and risk-taking behaviours (13).

A recent Cochrane review (15) of the evidence for the use of amphetamines to treat ADHD in adults found that there was sufficient evidence to suggest that amphetamines demonstrated greater effect size than placebo in reducing the symptom severity of ADHD in the short term only. It identified that the studies were of generally low quality with significant bias and short duration limiting the ability to demonstrate evidence for long-term efficacy of amphetamine treatment in adult ADHD and that it is an area that needs further investigation. Guidance from BAP cites the evidence supporting use of stimulant medication (methylphenidate and dexamfetamine) as well as non-stimulant (atomoxetine) as level '1a', that is to say that it is evidence-based on meta-analysis of randomised controlled trials, it does not comment on the quality of evidence from those trials (16).

Amphetamines were first synthesised in an attempt to create a substitute for adrenaline. The molecule in 3D modelling is almost indistinguishable from the monoamine neurotransmitters noradrenaline, adrenaline and dopamine. This is informative when considering the physiological effects of amphetamine as a drug of abuse and as stimulant medication to treat ADHD and narcolepsy (17). The psychopharmacology of amphetamines is complex with activity in a number of systems and brain circuits. The primary pharmacological effect is thought to be mediated by increased monoamine release. Amphetamines have been demonstrated to act in varying degrees as monoamine reuptake inhibitors and monoamine oxidase inhibitors and by these means to increase synaptic monoamines (17).

It may seem paradoxical that stimulants have been demonstrated to help in a disorder characterised by *hyper*-activity. In ADHD there are thought to be areas of hypofunction particularly in the pre-frontal cortex which lead to the poor planning and impulsivity seen in ADHD (13). Amphetamines have been demonstrated to increase monoamines, particularly dopamine and noradrenaline, within these circuits, which is believed to result in the clinical improvement demonstrated (16,17).

Q 3) A

Stimulant medications are only effective in 50–70% of individuals with ADHD (3,6). In addition the side effect profile of stimulant medications may mean that treatment is not tolerated. Finally, an individual may decide against stimulant medication because of stigma or the regulatory issues in elite sport (18). For these reasons it is important to consider non-pharmacological treatment options in consultation with the individual.

A recent Cochrane review (3) on the efficacy of CBT for the treatment of the core symptoms of ADHD in adults concluded that CBT plus pharmacological therapy demonstrated the best outcomes not only for ADHD symptomatology but also for treatment of co-morbid anxiety and depression. In contrast, NICE guidance (2018) (10) for managing ADHD in adults acknowledges the evidence base and makes the recommendation of pharmacotherapy as first-line treatment. The recommendation of non-pharmacological interventions (such as CBT) is present, but only for those who have made an 'informed choice not to have medication' (10).

Q 4) C

There has been significant debate over the use of stimulant medication in elite sport but a recent consensus statement by the IOC (9) has matched guidelines published by WADA accepting the need for stimulant medication in those with ADHD and significant functional impairment (5,18).

WADA publish an International Standard for TUEs (ISTUE) which outlines the process to athletes and anti-doping organisations for submitting, reviewing and monitoring TUEs (12).

The granting of a TUE can only occur if, by a balance of probabilities, the athlete can demonstrate that each of the following conditions is met, as defined by WADA (12):

1. The prohibited substance or prohibited method in question is needed to treat an acute or chronic medical condition, such that the athlete would experience a significant impairment to health if the prohibited substance or prohibited method were to be withheld
2. The therapeutic use of the prohibited substance or prohibited method is highly unlikely to produce any additional enhancement of performance beyond what might be anticipated by a return to the athlete's normal state of health following the treatment of the acute or chronic medical condition
3. There is no reasonable therapeutic alternative to the use of the prohibited substance or prohibited method
4. The necessity for the use of the prohibited substance or prohibited method is not a consequence, wholly or in part, of the prior use (without a TUE) of a substance or method which was prohibited at the time of such use

In 2018, UKAD launched a bespoke ADHD TUE policy in response to a marked increase in the number of TUEs granted for the use of stimulants to treat ADHD since 2014 (Figure 5.1) (18).

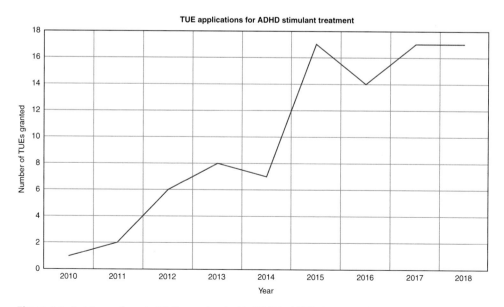

Figure 5.1. Incidence of granted TUEs associated with ADHD by UKAD since 2010. Data supplied by UKAD

A TUE application for the use of a stimulant medication to treat ADHD requires the submission of the specific ADHD TUE application form along with a report from a doctor (paediatrician, psychiatrist or other physician) specialising in the treatment of ADHD.

The UKAD ADHD TUE policy (19) requires that an accepted diagnostic schedule, e.g. Diagnostic Interview for Adult ADHD (DIVA) 2.0 (20), is submitted with all initial TUE applications to ensure the diagnosis is in accordance with the DSM-V criteria (5). It also stipulates that the report should include a copy of the full clinical assessment. A symptom severity rating scale matching the DSM-V guidelines, e.g. Adult ADHD Self-Report Scale (21), is also required for the initial application and for all subsequent renewal applications. Each renewal application should also be accompanied by a clinical report and update from a paediatrician, psychiatrist, or other clinician who specialises in the assessment and treatment of ADHD.

The UKAD ADHD TUE policy also introduced a mechanism for referring complex or borderline cases for a second opinion from an experienced psychiatrist serving on a register of preferred clinicians compiled by UKAD (19).

Compliance with anti-doping regulations is the responsibility of all competitive athletes (22). Full responsibilities regarding anti-doping regulations for athletes and their associates are available on the UKAD website (www.ukad.org.uk). Cycling-specific anti-doping information can be found on the website of the Cycling Anti-Doping Foundation: www.cadf.ch (23). The Anti-Doping Administration and Management System (ADAMS) is administered by WADA. ADAMS is a database that allows athletes and authorities to access and store information about testing results and any associated TUEs (12).

Although stimulants used to treat ADHD are only prohibited in-competition, there are many classes of drug on the WADA prohibited list that are prohibited at all times. This includes anabolic androgenic steroids, other hormones and metabolic modulators and agents affecting erythropoiesis. For this reason, athletes who are subject to anti-doping regulations must submit to random out-of-competition testing and ADAMS contains a 'Whereabouts' database to support this. Whereabouts technologies require the athlete to log exact locations per 60-minute slot with precise address and means of accessing them 24 hours a day, worldwide, in order that they can be available for random testing at any time (12). Compliance with the Whereabouts system is a regulatory requirement. Failure to log your locations can be seen as a violation of regulations and may be logged as a missed test. Three missed tests ('Whereabouts Failures') over 12 months can result in a ban from competing (22). As stated previously, stimulant medications used to treat ADHD fall into the WADA prohibited list under the category 'prohibited in-competition only' and can therefore be used legitimately out-of-competition without a TUE.

The testing regulations and requirements can be particularly taxing for athletes. Professional road cyclist Luke Rowe, when asked for comment on the practicalities of meeting anti-doping regulations, stated that:

> As riders we recognise the need to be fully aware and compliant with the WADA regulations and 'whereabouts' criteria; however, as a professional cyclist in a very busy world-wide racing calendar, it takes a lot of time, concentration and energy to make sure I am fully compliant with my travel plans, flights, hotel accommodation and time differences across the globe! Even changes outside my designated 60 minutes I have to be aware of, and make sure I can get back to my testing if needed within 60 minutes.

Q 5) D

One meta-analysis of adolescent athletes aged 15–19 identified rates of ADHD at double those of the general population (24) while a narrative review commented on the scarcity of studies in elite sport but concluded that ADHD prevalence rates may be higher in certain sports (25). Approximately 8.4% of Major League Baseball (MLB) players in the 2017–2018 season in the US are reported as having a TUE for ADHD stimulant medication (26). Hyun Han et al. (25) cite reasons why this figure is likely to be an underestimate of actual rates of the disorder in the population; these include the fact that the threshold for receiving a TUE for ADHD in elite sport is much higher than that required for diagnosis and medication in the general population. Further, they suggest that given the stigma and resistance to stimulant medication in elite sport the 8.4% represents only those who actually required stimulant medication for their ADHD and the figure for those with ADHD who either chose not to go through the stresses of the TUE application process or who responded well to psychological interventions or non-stimulant medication is therefore likely to be much higher (25).

The reasons why ADHD might be more prevalent in some sports are unclear. It is presumed that it is a multi-factorial association. It is acknowledged that sport and physical activity are encouraged in children with the disorder given their levels of hyperactivity and therefore they may be pushed into this arena. There is also a suggestion that some attributes central to the disorder itself such as risk-taking behaviour, impulsivity and quick thinking might lead to a predisposition for success within certain sports (18,25,27). Others have postulated that ADHD may negatively affect performance but only in some sporting activities such as equestrian events and in certain football and baseball positions (28).

> **Summary of the Chapter and the Topics Covered**
>
> - Diagnosis and management of ADHD in sport
> - Risk factors associated with ADHD along with co-morbid depression and anxiety
> - The anti-doping status of medications used in the management of ADHD
> - The required standard of supporting medical evidence to be contained within a TUE application for the use of stimulant medication for ADHD
> - The importance of considering non-pharmacological management of psychiatric illness particularly in elite sport

Acknowledgements

We would like to thank Samuel Pool, Medical Programmes Officer at UKAD, for support with Figure 5.1 and data interpretation of the latest UK TUE data.

References

1. American Psychiatric Association. *Diagnostic and Statistical Manual of Mental Disorders (DSM-5)*. Washington, DC. American Psychiatric Publishing. 2013.

2. World Health Organization. *International Classification of Diseases*. ICD-10. Available from: https://icd.who.int/

3. Lopez PL, Torrente FM, Ciapponi A, Lischinsky AG, Cetkovich-Bakmas M, Rojas JI, et al. Cognitive-behavioural interventions for attention deficit hyperactivity disorder (ADHD) in adults. *Cochrane Database of Systematic Reviews*. 2018;3:Art.No.CD010840. DOI:10.1002/14651858.CD010840.pub2 www.cochranelibrary.com

4. Kessler R, Adle L, Barklay R, Biederman J, Conners K, Farone S, et al. Patterns and predictors of ADHD persistence into adulthood: Results from the National Comorbidity Survey Replication. *Biol Psychiatry*. 2005;57(11):1442–51.

5. World Anti-Doping Agency (WADA). *Attention Deficit Hyperactivity Disorder (ADHD) in Children and Adults* . TUEC guidelines: Medical information to support the decisions of TUE committees – Version 6.0. 2017. Available from: www.wada-ama.org/en/resources/therapeutic-use-exemption-tue/medical-information-to-support-the-decisions-of-tuecs-adhd

6. Kooij SJJ, et al. European consensus statement on diagnosis and treatment of adult ADHD: The European Network Adult ADHD. *BMC Psychiatry*. 2010; 10:67.

7. Simon V, Czobor P, Bálint S, Mészáros Á, Bitter I. Prevalence and correlates of adult attention-deficit hyperactivity disorder: Meta-analysis. *BJ Psychiatry*. 2009;194(3):204–11. doi:10.1192/bjp.bp.107.048827.

8. Royal College of Psychiatrists. *ADHD in Adults: Good Practice Guidelines*. Royal College of Psychiatrists in Scotland special interest group in ADHD. 2017. Available from: www.rcpsych.ac.uk

9. Reardon C, Hainline B, Aron CM, et al. Mental health in elite athletes: International Olympic Committee consensus statement (2019). *Br J Sports Med*. 2019;53:667–99.

10. National Institute for Health and Clinical Excellence. *Attention Deficit Hyperactivity Disorder: Diagnosis and Management*. NICE Guideline 87. NICE. 2018. Available from: www.nice.org.uk

11. British National Formulary. Website: bnf.nice.org.uk. 2019.

12. World Anti-Doping Agency. Website: www.wada-ama.org. 2019.

13. Rosler M, Casas M, Konofal E, Buitelaar J. Attention deficit hyperactivity disorder in adults. *The World Journal of Biological Psychiatry*. 2010;11:684–98.

14. Driver and Vehicle Licensing Authority. Attention deficit hyperactivity disorder (ADHD) and driving. 2019. Available from: www.gov.uk/adhd-and-driving.

15. Castells X, Blanco-Silvente L, Cunill R. Amphetamines for attention deficit hyperactivity disorder (ADHD) in adults. *Cochrane Database of Systematic Reviews*.2018;8.Art.No.CD007813. DOI:10.1002/14651858.CD007813.pub3.www.cochranelibrary.com

16. Bolea-Alamañac B, Nutt DJ, Adamou M, Asherson P, Bazire S, Coghill D, et al. Evidence-based guidelines for the pharmacological management of attention deficit hyperactivity disorder: Update on recommendations from the British Association for Psychopharmacology. *J Psychopharmacol*. 2014;28(3):179–203.

17. Heal D, Smith S, Gosden J, Nutt D; Amphetamine, past and present: A pharmacological and clinical perspective. *Journal of Psychopharmacology*. 2013;27(6):479–96.

18. Pool S, Currie, A. Anti-doping considerations for treating athletes with ADHD. *ADHD in Practice*. 2018;10(3).

19. United Kingdom Anti-Doping. *ADHD TUE Policy*. QAP10-05 V1.2. 2019. Available from: www.ukad.org.uk

20. Kooij J. *Diagnostic Interview for ADHD in Adults 2.0 (DIVA 2.0): Diagnostic Assessment and Treatment*. Amsterdam, the Netherlands: Pearson Assessment and Information BV; 2010. www.divacentre.eu.

21. Adult ADHD Self-Report Scale (ASRS-v1.1). 2019. Available from: https://add.org/wp-content/uploads/2015/03/adhd-questionnaire-ASRS111.pdf

22. United Kingdom Anti-Doping. Website: www.ukad.org.uk. 2019.

23. Cycling Anti-Doping Foundation. Website: www.cadf.ch. 2019.

24. Garner A, Hansen A, Baxley C, Ross M; The use of stimulant medication to treat attention-deficit/hyperactivity disorder in elite athletes: A performance and health perspective. *Sports Med*. (2018);48:507–12.

25. Han DH, McDuff D, Thompson D, Hitchcock M, Reardon C, Hainline B.

Attention-deficit/hyperactivity disorder in elite athletes: A narrative review. *Br J of Sports Med.* 2019;53:741–5.

26. Martin T. *Public Report of Major League Baseball's Joint Drug Prevention and Treatment Program.* 2018. Available from: www.mlb.com/documents/3/8/2/30 1315382/IPA_2018_Public_ Report_ 1130 18. pdf

27. Reardon C, Factor R. Considerations in the use of stimulants in sport. *Sports Med.* 2016;46:611–17

28. Conant-Norville DO, Tofler IR. Attention deficit/hyperactivity disorder and psychopharmacologic treatments in the athlete. *Clinics in Sports Medicine.* 2005;24 (4):829–43. https://doi.org/10.1016/j .csm.2005.05.007

6

Football: Alcohol and Barriers to Support

Amit Mistry, Steve Peters and Robin Chatterjee
Athlete expert advisor: David Cotterill

A small aspect of football culture has an enmeshed history with alcohol and can create an environment where harmful alcohol consumption is promoted. As a result, both current and former professional footballers are at risk. Alcohol-related psychiatric assessments need to serially assess severity, risk and social function and manage any co-morbid physical or mental health conditions. Following these assessments, a personalised biopsychosocial care plan should be agreed. A sports psychiatrist must understand how alcohol misuse presents within the elite football environment and how patient motivation towards behaviour change is central to recovery.

Background

AS is a 23-year-old defender for an English professional football team. Thirteen months ago he injured his right anterior cruciate ligament (ACL). This required reconstruction and he was sidelined for eight months. Two months after returning to play he re-injured the same ACL and has since been receiving further rehabilitative physiotherapy. He admitted struggling with the injury and was concerned about his future as a footballer.

Over the last month, team members had become increasingly concerned by his increasing alcohol consumption and change in behaviour. His temper appeared short and he seemed to have lost his footballing 'drive'. He eventually agreed for the club doctor to refer him to a sports psychiatrist with addiction treatment expertise. A copy of the psychiatric consultation is outlined below.

Presenting Complaint

'The lads have got me worried about my boozing, so I should try to get some help.'

History of Presenting Complaint

A admitted to a three-month history of binge drinking three times/week. Each session averaged four pints of 4.0% beer with two double whisky shots (13 units x 3 = 39 units/week) at post-match socials and during mid-week snooker sessions with other players. He denied requiring alcohol to reduce any withdrawal symptoms, although had noticed that he needs larger amounts of alcohol to have an intoxicating effect. He reported being 'too shy' and could only 'have a good time' when drinking. The thought of speaking up at team meetings made him feel 'panicky'.

A's alcohol consumption had gradually increased over the last year and he was fearful that this might turn into a daily habit. He first drank beer on a school trip at the age of 14. He has never drunk regularly, particularly once he secured his first professional contract. Childhood memories of his father's aggression under the influence of alcohol used to act as a deterrent. Increased drinking started after his first injury 13 months ago. Since then his volume and frequency of alcohol use had slowly increased. He had never sought alcohol support before and presumed it was largely up to him to 'sort it out'.

A wanted to reduce and ultimately stop his alcohol bingeing as he knew this could have a negative impact on injury recovery and ultimately performance on the pitch. Through his own initiative, he had contemplated doing online educational courses in his free time that would help 'boost his CV' and provide a distraction away from 'going out and boozing it up'.

There were no reported symptoms of depression, psychosis, generalised anxiety or post-traumatic stress disorder (PTSD) following his knee injury.

Past Psychiatric History

There was no past psychiatric history.

Family History

Father had a 'drinking problem' but never sought professional help.

He had two elder brothers with no reported mental health conditions.

Past Medical History

Recurrent right knee ACL injury with surgical correction.

Medication

No known drug allergies.

Paracetamol 1g as required for pain, maximum four times daily.

Never prescribed any psychotropic medication.

Social History

A lived alone in his own home. He had no reported financial concerns and had already paid off his mortgage. He passed his driving test at the age of 17 and drove his own car. Most of his family members still lived in Glasgow although remained in regular contact with him.

He had tried cocaine on two occasions since being injured but denied this being a regular habit. He denied smoking cigarettes or using vape devices.

Personal History

A denied any reported complications at birth and achieved normal childhood developmental milestones. He enjoyed attending first school and was popular within his year. A denied any personal childhood adversities (such as bullying or abuse) but remembered times when his father would drink alcohol and get into heated arguments with his mother. He did not wish to discuss this in any further detail.

During his teenage years, he worked very hard to become a professional footballer and admitted that he had neglected his formal education. He obtained a National Vocational Qualification (NVQ) Level 1 in Sports and Recreation but had never worked outside playing professional football. At the age of 16, he moved away from his family home in Glasgow to train with his club's academy side in London. At the age of 18, he became the first Scottish youth player to sign a professional contract for the club based in London. He was now nearing the end of his five-year professional contract.

A was single, having recently broken up from a heterosexual relationship. Since then he has had several, 'uncharacteristic, one-night stands' and felt severe guilt the next morning.

Pre-Morbid Personality

A described himself as always being 'quiet' but 'popular' and put this down to being a good footballer at school. A believed his mood had 'dipped' over the last month.

Forensic History

Thirteen months ago, he was arrested for common assault on a stranger while intoxicated on a team night out. He was given a fine and community order although there was no other involvement with police or the criminal justice system. He denied any history of sexual misconduct or drug-related offences.

Collateral History

He refused family member involvement although reported that his brother had become worried about his recent drinking behaviour.

Mental State Examination

A presented as a 23-year-old Caucasian male, who was wearing his team tracksuit and was kempt in appearance. He was mobilising with crutches and had a right-sided antalgic gait. He was hesitant initially, pleasant in interaction and demonstrated good eye contact. There was no evidence of psychomotor retardation and normal speech pattern in all modalities (rate, tone and volume). He communicated his frustrations regarding his injury in a congruent manner. He did not present with any symptoms suggestive of an acute depressive episode, generalised anxiety or PTSD. There was no evidence of disordered thought. He believed that his new alcohol binges were linked to boredom and uncertainty about his playing career. A was unsure whether he should retire from professional football and was disappointed that his coach had not discussed this with him. He remained fearful that if he sought help from management he would be perceived as 'weak and attention-seeking. I don't want to give them more reasons to drop me from the squad'.

A possessed relatively good insight into his harmful alcohol consumption and had responded to external prompts to seek external alcohol support. He wished to reduce his problematic alcohol binge behaviour and was willing to engage with treatment options available to him. He was at the action stage of the transtheoretical change model (1) and had outlined his plans to address his alcohol consumption. He presented with both intrinsic (e.g. own concerns about behaviour, detrimental impact on injury recovery, his footballer identity, remembering how alcohol affected his father growing up) and extrinsic motivators (e.g. concerns by family and team members) to control his alcohol misuse. This was his first presentation for alcohol support and he scored 30/30 on MMSE.

Risk Assessment

Self: No evidence of suicide ideation, active suicide or self-harm plans. His current alcohol consumption potentially placed him at risk of accidents while under the influence e.g. risk of violence, disinhibited behaviour such as unprotected sexual intercourse leading to sexually transmitted infections along with long-term physical health risks if current pattern not addressed.

Others: No expressed risks to others although historic assault on a member of the public while under the influence of alcohol.

Protective factors: A was well motivated to address his alcohol consumption and engage in professional support.

Investigations

No reported abnormalities on physical examination or blood screening (including normal LFTs and clotting).

No acute alcohol withdrawal on Clinical Institute Withdrawal Assessment for Alcohol (CIWA-Ar). CIWA-Ar (revised version) is a sensitive 10-item scale used to assess and manage patients in alcohol withdrawal.

Case Formulation

A presented as a 23-year-old, male, single professional footballer with a severe alcohol use disorder, which had escalated following his second knee injury around three months ago. His alcohol consumption had escalated within the last year.

A's father had a history of alcohol misuse, which suggested a hereditary predisposing risk (genetic loading). Perpetuating factors included being low in mood, 'bored', frustrated with his injury, associated pain and the uncertainty regarding his future footballing career. He had become isolated from family support and socialised in environments where excess alcohol consumption was often encouraged. He reported how alcohol consumption around the team environment had become habitual and how he often felt 'shy' if not drinking alcohol. On review of protective factors, A was motivated towards behaviour change and had good insight into the detrimental effects of alcohol on his playing status.

Plan

- A was allocated an alcohol key worker who would work with him on a 1:1 basis and explore suitable psychosocial interventions for him
- A was provided with a leaflet listing local alcohol support groups and a mobile app that will help him track his alcohol consumption
- A wanted time to decide whether he would like the clinic letter to be sent to his team doctor. He was reminded that he could seek further '24/7' confidential support from the PFA. The PFA provides this helpline for both current and former PFA members. Any

player, concerned family member or friend can email them on wellbeing@thepfa.co.uk or call 07500 000 777

- A was offered a further follow-up appointment in the outpatient clinic. The next review in two weeks' time would determine whether pharmacological treatment for alcohol misuse may be a suitable option for him. The appointment would also be used to review his engagement with support groups and any changes in his pattern of alcohol use. He would also update his psychiatrist on whether he would like his team doctor to have a written copy of the assessment

Questions

Q 1   If the Psychiatrist used the Alcohol Use Disorders Identification Test Consumption (AUDIT-C) screening tool, what would A have scored?
   A. Scored 0–4, indicates low risk
   B. Scored 5–7, indicates increasing risk
   C. Scored 8–10, indicates higher risk
   D. Scored 11–12, indicates possible alcohol dependence
   E. No risk identified

Q 2   What treatment will be offered to him following the Alcohol Use Disorder (AUD) diagnosis?
   A. DBT
   B. Acamprosate 666mg three times a day
   C. Psychosocial interventions with or without medication for relapse prevention
   D. Psychosocial interventions with medication for assisted alcohol withdrawal only
   E. SSRI

Q 3   A reflected on his recent drinking behaviour and commented on how he meets retired team-mates with worse alcohol consumption than him. He asked whether being retired from football increases mental health risks. What would your response be?
   A. There is some evidence suggesting that retired footballers have a greater risk of common mental disorders (CMD) including alcohol misuse compared to current professional footballers
   B. There is robust, level-1 evidence (high) confirming this observation
   C. No, current professional footballers definitely have higher rates of alcohol misuse than retired players
   D. There is no evidence to suggest that recurrent injury status is linked with CMD
   E. No, being athletes they are at much lower risk of experiencing CMD than the general population

Q 4   One week after the team doctor's consultation, a worker at the football club witnessed A driving his car erratically around the training ground. There were no reported casualties from the incident. He apparently presented as intoxicated while exiting his vehicle. The team doctor was informed. What should be his or her next steps?
   A. Ensure that A's thoughts on the incident are urgently explored at his next CBT session
   B. Arrange a random alcohol breath test

C. Inform A that you now have a duty of care to inform his parents about the incident

D. Accept that this was a likely one-off incident and forget about it

E. Arrange to meet with A as soon as practically possible, tell him to stop driving and inform the DVLA about his alcohol misuse

Q 5 Recently, there is greater awareness in English football of the risks of alcohol misuse and how to access support. (True or False?)

Answers

Q 1) D

AUDIT-C (Table 6.1A) is a widely used and validated screening tool (3). Alternatives include the brief CAGE questionnaire although this is most helpful in identifying the extreme end of severe alcohol misuse (4). Screening alone is not enough to review alcohol misuse but can provide a useful opportunity to deliver brief therapeutic interventions.

Table 6.1A AUDIT-C initial screening questions and scoring guide

Question	Scoring System				
	0	1	2	3	4
How often do you have a drink containing alcohol?	Never	Monthly or less	2 to 4 times per month	2 to 3 times per week	4 or more times per week
How many units of alcohol do you drink on a typical day when you are drinking?	0–2	3–4	5–6	7–9	10 +
How often have you had 6 or more units if female, or 8 or more if male, on a single occasion in the last year?	Never	Less than monthly	Monthly	Weekly	Daily or almost daily

Scoring	Alcohol Use Disorder
0–4	Low risk
5+	POSITIVE Screen
5–7	Increasing risk
8–10	Higher risk
11–12	Possible dependence

Any score above 5 suggests a higher risk for alcohol disorder and A's score of 11 indicated possible alcohol dependence. In those identified as being at risk, the full AUDIT tool should then be completed. This reduces 'false-positive' risk and identifies higher-risk patients who need more than brief alcohol intervention and advice, e.g. those with AUDIT scores over 20 (possible alcohol dependence). Clinicians often start with the AUDIT-C tool and may supplement this with the AUDIT tool dependent on the patient's initial score. Table 6.1B outlines the AUDIT questionnaire with scoring breakdown (3):

Table 6.1B Remaining assessment questions with complete AUDIT scoring guide.

Questions	Scoring System				
	0	1	2	3	4
How often during the last year have you found that you were not able to stop drinking once you had started?	Never	Less than monthly	Monthly	Weekly	Daily or almost daily
How often during the last year have you failed to do what was normally expected from you because of your drinking?	Never	Less than monthly	Monthly	Weekly	Daily or almost daily
How often during the last year have you needed an alcoholic drink in the morning to get yourself going after a heavy drinking session?	Never	Less than monthly	Monthly	Weekly	Daily or almost daily
How often during the last year have you had a feeling of guilt or remorse after drinking?	Never	Less than monthly	Monthly	Weekly	Daily or almost daily
How often during the last year have you been unable to remember what happened the night before because you had been drinking?	Never	Less than monthly	Monthly	Weekly	Daily or almost daily
Have you or somebody else been injured as a result of your drinking?	No		Yes, but not in the last year		Yes, during the last year
Has a relative or friend, doctor or other health worker been concerned about your drinking or suggested that you cut down?	No		Yes, but not in the last year		Yes, during the last year

Scoring	Alcohol Use Disorder
0–7	Low risk
8–15	Increasing risk (hazardous drinking)
16–19	Higher risk (harmful drinking)
20+	Possible dependence

A reported that he has never struggled to stop alcohol consumption while drinking (0 points) or forgotten events from a previous night (0 points) but admitted to missing a recent meeting due to a 'hangover' (1 point). He denied requiring alcohol to control alcohol withdrawal symptoms in the morning but does infrequently experience alcohol-related guilt (1 point). He assaulted someone 13 months ago while being intoxicated (2 points) and accepted team member concerns regarding his drinking (4 points). His score of 19 out of 40 on the full 10 screening questions suggests harmful drinking.

Q 2) C

A presented with a moderately harmful AUD. Most patients aim for total abstinence although some opt for moderation instead. A step-wise, comprehensive plan must manage any acute alcohol intoxication, treat withdrawal symptoms and address any co-morbid psychiatric and/or medical conditions (5). All treatment goals should be transparent and supported by an allocated key worker.

Conventional psychosocial therapies for alcohol misuse include self-help and stepped recovery programmes, e.g. alcohol support group therapy for alcohol misuse can be useful for elite athletes, although barriers to care include busy training schedules, low mental health literacy, previous negative experiences seeking treatment and perceived stigma (6,7,8).

Brief interventions of 1–4 sessions last up to 60 minutes and are delivered by health care professionals who can help patients reduce their alcohol intake. However, younger, less educated patients with lower motivation towards intervention are at higher risk of treatment drop out (9,10).

Psychological treatments include CBT, behavioural therapy or behavioural couples' therapy. Weekly therapy sessions last 10–45 minutes over a twelve-week period and are underpinned by non-judgemental, motivational interviewing (MI) techniques designed to identify ambivalence towards treatment and explore personal problems related to alcohol. MI is based on 'patient empathy', 'supporting self-efficacy' and 'developing discrepancy' by highlighting the differences between the patient's current and desired behaviour and 'rolling with resistance'. Rolling with resistance reflects on patient viewpoints in a sensitive, non-confrontational manner (11). The athlete's stage of change along with motivation towards intervention is paramount for recovery (12,13). Athletes tend to be well-motivated individuals and well placed to benefit from treatment interventions (13). Again, football training commitments may impact on their ability to attend regular, therapy.

Pharmacotherapy is reserved for those with higher levels of alcohol misuse. Medication can be used to manage withdrawal, cravings or co-morbid mental illness or symptoms, e.g. depression, anxiety or insomnia. Pharmacological options to manage persistent, debilitating cravings include naltrexone, acamprosate and disulfiram. These have a well-established, moderate efficacy and can be initiated once alcohol withdrawal is treated (12,14).

Naltrexone is an opiate antagonist which prevents opioid receptor stimulation and reduces dopamine release from the ventral tegmental area (VTA), a key part of the brain's reward circuitry. It possesses a small–moderate effect size (ES, 0.1–0.5) (12). Athletes must not be taking opiate analgesics with this medication as its antagonist profile may induce unpleasant opiate withdrawal symptoms.

Acamprosate is a N-methyl D-aspartate receptor antagonist and positive modulator of the γ-aminobutyric acid (GABA-A) receptor. Its proposed neuroprotective action normalises glutaminergic systems during early alcohol abstinence (12). It is generally well tolerated and more effective than placebo at increasing abstinence, particularly when patients possess greater levels of motivation (12,15,16).

Disulfiram, a GABA analogue, is offered when there are contraindications to the two options above. It is an aversive agent and can be prescribed 24 hours after the last consumed drink. There is limited evidence suggesting therapeutic superiority over placebo, and it is most effective when used as an adjunct to psychotherapeutic interventions (12). There is no evidence that combining naltrexone, acamprosate or disulfiram together enhances therapeutic response (5,17).

Off-licence pharmacological options such as ondansetron (a selective serotonergic, 5-HT3 antagonist) may be particularly effective in younger patients (<25 years old) with early-onset alcohol disorder (14). Antagonism of 5-HT3 receptor sites within mesolimbic brain areas, e.g. VTA, nucleus accumbens (NA) or amygdala, may reduce alcohol self-administration and some of its subjective effects (18). Also, flexible, electronic forms of counselling (e.g. e-CBT) may be more suited for frequent travellers such as footballers. Table 6.2 summarises the available management options for AUD severities based on AUDIT scores (3,5).

Table 6.2 Available management options for AUD severities based on AUDIT scores

AUDIT Score	Alcohol Use Disorder	Management
0–7	Indicates low risk	Nil
8–15	Indicates increasing risk (hazardous drinking)	Simple structured advice CBT, behaviour couples' therapy Social network- and environment-based therapies
16–19	Indicates higher risk (harmful drinking)	Brief interventions and follow up CBT, behaviour couples' therapy Social network- and environment-based therapies
20+	Indicates possible dependence	Referral on to specialist alcohol services Medically assisted withdrawal/detoxification (chlordiazepoxide or diazepam regime as inpatient or outpatient dependent on severity) Thiamine (oral PO or intramuscular IM) to prevent Wernicke's encephalopathy or Korsakoff's syndrome Pharmacotherapy should be offered in conjunction with psychosocial interventions.

Q 3) A

Elite athletes consume alcohol for similar reasons to those of the general population (13). Higher use in team sports may be linked to the subjective need to enhance team spirit, which can lead to team-mates normalising and over-estimating each other's consumption. Other factors include permissive attitudes towards higher alcohol consumption within the extended sport's family (6,19).

Severe or recurrent injuries, especially those linked with early, involuntary retirement, can predispose athletes to CMD such as depression, anxiety, distress and adverse health behaviours (e.g. alcohol, smoking and poor nutrition) (20). Alcohol binge-drinking rates are higher in elite professional athletes (compared to general population) and increase with transitions into retirement (21). A series of small, pilot, cross-sectional studies by the Fédération Internationale des Associations de Footballeurs Professionnels (FIFPro) in 149 current and 104 former professional footballers indicated increased rates of adverse alcohol behaviour (AUDIT-C score >5) (32% vs. 19%) in retired compared to current footballers (22). Also, a recent meta-analysis demonstrated that former athletes from various sports have higher alcohol misuse rates compared to current athletes (21% vs. 19% respectively) (23).

Alcohol misuse in former professionals could be secondary to transitioning distress, 'self-treatment' for previous injury pain and possessing a lack of alternative, structured activities (23). Further retirement stressors include low social support, financial problems, lack of career planning and limited educational opportunity. It has been proposed that footballers should be offered mental health self-awareness and career-exit examinations to support post-retirement wellbeing (20,21). Regardless of playing status, sports clinicians need to reiterate that excessive alcohol consumption possesses 'ergolytic' effects (the opposite of performance enhancing effects) such as insomnia, dehydration, weight gain, impaired psychomotor skills, injury risk and slower healing rate (6,21,24).

Psychiatric Emergency Box

Acute alcohol withdrawal syndrome can be life threatening and is not always directly related to the intake amount (25,26). Table 6.3 outlines the common manifestations of alcohol withdrawal syndrome.

Table 6.3 Manifestations of alcohol withdrawal syndrome (adapted from the Maudsley Prescribing Guidelines) (26)

Severity of alcohol withdrawal	Manifestations	Usual timing of onset after last drink
Mild	Agitation, irritability, anxiety Tremor of hands, eyelids, tongue Sweating Nausea/vomiting/diarrhoea Fever Tachycardia General malaise	Onset at 3–12 hours Peak at 24–48 hours Duration up to 14 days
Severe	Generalised seizures	12–18 hours

Withdrawal symptoms manifest 4–12 hours after the last drink and peak at 10–30 hours. Signs and symptoms are monitored using the Clinical Institute Withdrawal Assessment for Alcohol (CIWA-Ar) scale (Figure 6.1) (2). Treatment for central nervous system (CNS) irritability includes short-term as-required benzodiazepines such as chlordiazepoxide followed by a lengthier fixed-dose or symptom-triggered withdrawal-reducing regimen. A typical fixed-dose reducing regime is over a 5–7 day period and is prescribed based on the baseline chlordiazepoxide dose, which is determined by CIWA-Ar withdrawal score (2, 26). Alcohol withdrawal treatment interventions are a combination of supportive medical care, pharmacology for neuroadaptation reversal and thiamine supplementation. Again, the level of medical monitoring, medication dosage and treatment setting (home, community or inpatient setting) is dependent on withdrawal severity (26).

Delirium tremens (DTs) is a MEDICAL EMERGENCY and occurs in around 5% of alcohol withdrawal states. This occurs when chronic alcohol use is suddenly stopped or significantly reduced and the brain's neurochemical compensatory response results in sympathetic overdrive (autonomic hyperexcitability). This may result in cardiorespiratory collapse or cardiac arrhythmia and can be fatal. If untreated, mortality rate is 15–20% but with appropriate intervention reduces down to 1% (27). DTs presents with fluctuating consciousness, disorientation, short-term memory loss, psychomotor agitation and hallucinations (visual, auditory and tactile). Its onset is typically 2–3 days after the last alcohol

Heart Rate _____

Blood Pressure _____

Figure 6.1 Clinical Institute Withdrawal Assessment for Alcohol (CIWA-Ar) scale (2)

NAUSEA AND VOMITING -- "Do you feel sick to your stomach? Have you vomited?"
0 Mild nausea with no vomiting
1
2
3
4 Intermittent nausea with dry heaves
5
6
7 Constant nausea, frequent dry heaves and vomiting

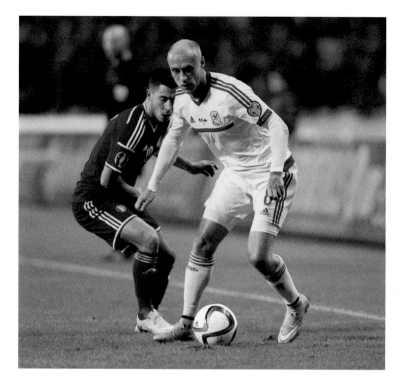

1 Footballer David Cotterill. Photo provided by David Cotterill (co-author, expert athlete advisor)

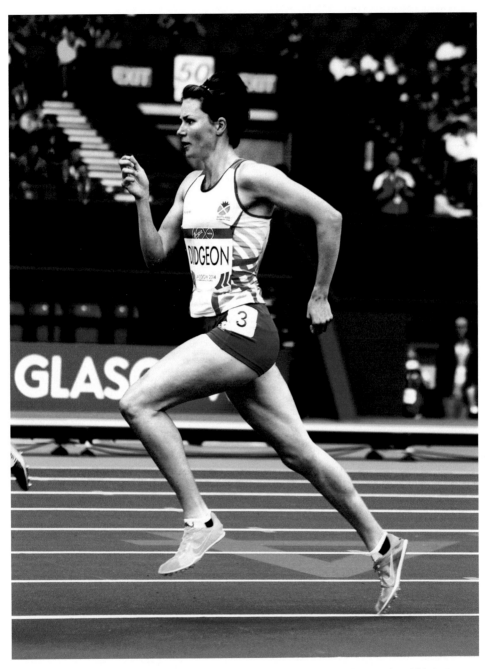

2 Endurance runner Emily Dudgeon. Photo provided by Mark Shearman (Sports photographer, Athletics Images athleticsimages.com)

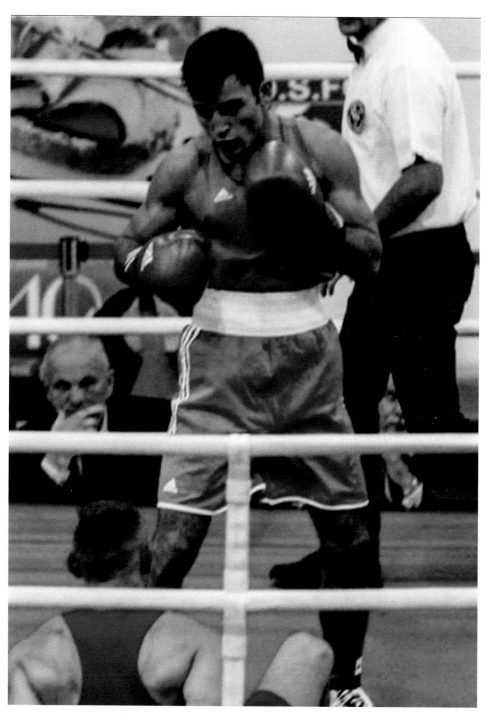

3 Boxer Cyrus Pattinson. Photo provided by Chris Connolly (English Institute of Sport Performance Analyst)

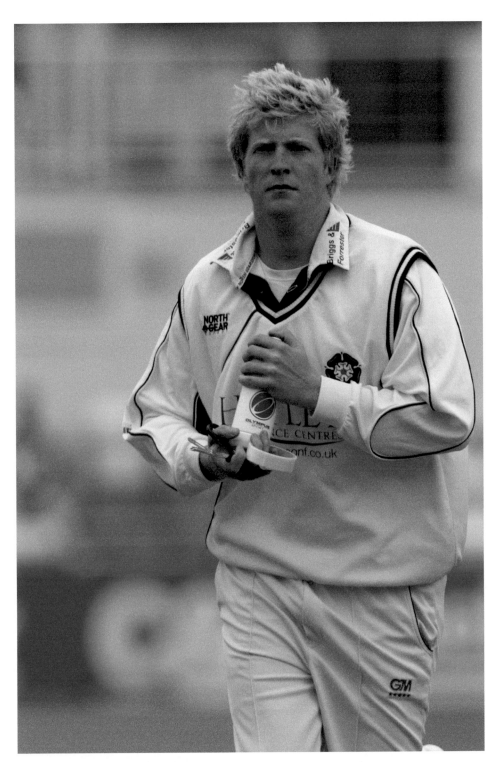

4 Cricketer Patrick Foster. Photo provided by Patrick Foster (co-author, expert athlete advisor)

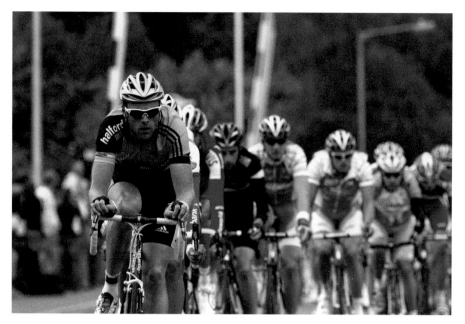

5 Cyclists in competition. Photo provided by Alan Currie (author)

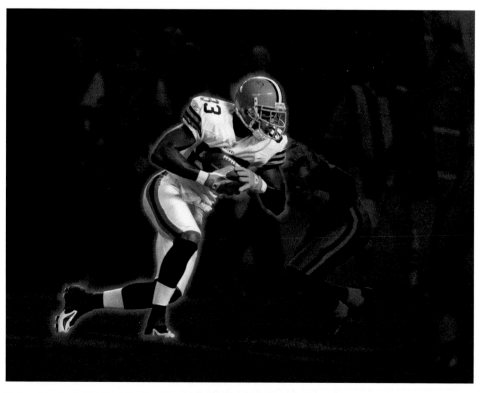

6 American footballer Steve Sanders. Photo provided by Steve Sanders (co-author, expert athlete advisor)

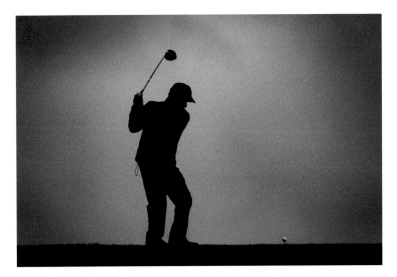

7 Golfer. Photo provided by Campbell Skinner (Photographer, Campbell Skinner Photography)

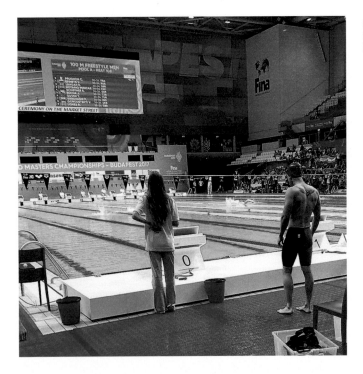

8 Swimmer Omar Hussain. Photo provided by Omar Hussain (GB Masters swimmer)

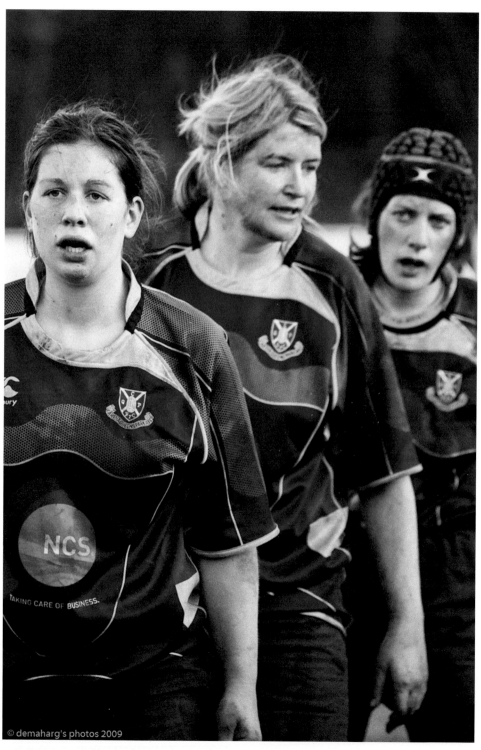

© demaharg's photos 2009

9 Rugby players. Photo provided by Campbell Skinner (Photographer, Campbell Skinner Photography)

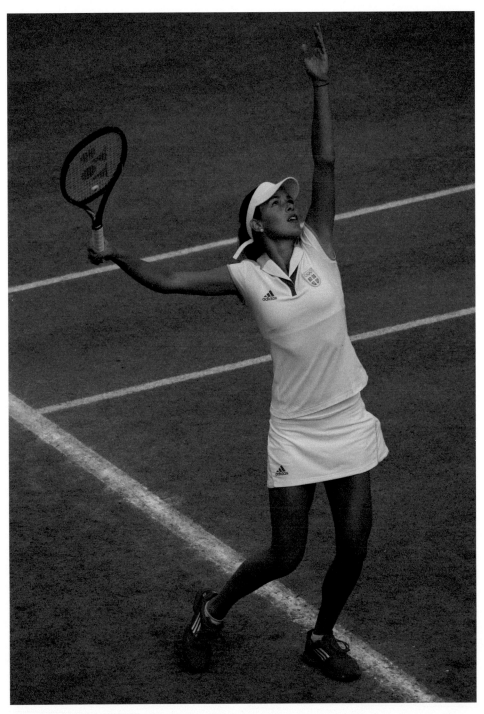

10 Tennis player Ana Ivanovic. Photo provided by Zoë Reeve (Photographer, Unsplash)

TACTILE DISTURBANCES -- Ask "Have you any itching, pins and needles sensations, any burning, any numbness, or do you feel bugs crawling on or under your skin?"
0 None
1 Very mild itching, pins and needles, burning or numbness
2 Mild itching, pins and needles, burning or numbness
3 Moderate itching, pins and needles, burning or numbness
4 Moderately severe hallucinations
5 Severe hallucinations
6 Extremely severe hallucinations
7 Continuous hallucinations

AUDITORY DISTURBANCES -- Ask "Are you more aware of sounds around you? Are they harsh? Do they frighten you? Are you hearing anything that is disturbing to you? Are you hearing things you know are not there?"
0 Not present
1 Very mild harshness or ability to frighten
2 Mild harshness or ability to frighten
3 Moderate harshness or ability to frighten
4 Moderately severe hallucinations
5 Severe hallucinations
6 Extremely severe hallucinations
7 Continuous hallucinations

TREMOR -- Arms extended and fingers spread apart.
0 No tremor
1 Not visible, but can be felt
2
3
4 Moderate, with patient's arms
5
6
7 Severe, even with arms not extended

PAROXYSMAL SWEATS
0 No sweat visible
1 Barely perceptible sweating, palms moist fingertip to fingertip
2
3
4 Beads of sweat obviously on forehead
5
6
7 Drenching sweats

Figure 6.1-1 (Cont.)

ANXIETY -- Ask "Do you feel nervous?"
0 No anxiety, at ease
1 Mildly anxious
2
3
4 Moderately anxious, or guarded, so anxiety is inferred
5
6
7 Equivalent to acute panic states as seen in severe delirium or acute schizophrenic reactions

HEADACHE, FULLNESS IN HEAD -- Ask "Does your head feel different? Does it feel like there is a band around your head?" Do not rate for dizziness or lightheadedness. Otherwise, rate severity
0 Not present
1 Very mild
2 Mild
3 Moderate
4 Moderately severe
5 Severe
6 Very severe
7 Extremely severe

AGITATION
0 Normal activity
1 Somewhat more than normal activity
2
3
4 Moderately fidgety and restless
5
6
7 Paces back and forth during most of the interview, or constantly thrashes about

ORIENTATION AND CLOUDING OF SENSORIUM -- Ask "What day is this? Where are we? Who am I?"
0 Oriented and can do serial additions
1 Cannot do serial additions or is uncertain about date
2 Disoriented for date by no more than 2 calendar days
3 Disoriented for date by more than 2 calendar days
4 Disoriented for place/or person

Figure 6.1-2 (Cont.)

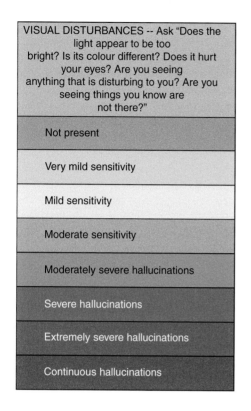

Figure 6.1-3 (Cont.)

drink (16). Treatment involves a further benzodiazepine treatment course led by a medical clinician with expertise in this area.

Additional treatments for known or suspected chronic alcohol misuse include intramuscular (IM) Pabrinex © to treat Wernicke's encephalopathy (WE). This is an acute neuropsychiatric condition caused by severe thiamine deficiency. Any patient undergoing detoxification who experiences confusion, memory impairment, ataxia, hypothermia, hypotension, ocular motility disorders or unconsciousness has a presumptive diagnosis of WE. If left untreated, WE can progress to irreversible Korsakoff syndrome. This results in memory impairment, confabulation, confusion and personality changes. Common somatic complaints during alcohol withdrawal include dehydration, nausea, vomiting, diarrhoea, skin itching and pain and can be managed using basic pharmacological measures (26).

Q 4) E

This incident may have required a breach in confidentiality, although not necessarily to his nearest relative. General Medical Council guidance is that doctors can breach patient confidentiality if there is a greater need to protect the general public or under the duress of legal proceedings (www.gmc-uk.org/ethical-guidance/ethical-guidance-for-doctors/con fidentiality—patients-fitness-to-drive-and-reporting-concerns-to-the-dvla-or-dva).   This may strain the therapeutic relationship between patient and clinician (28).

In the above scenario, the doctor should meet with A as soon as practically possible and advise him to stop driving. His alcohol misuse is impacting on his fitness to drive and he should be offered the opportunity to disclose this information to the DVLA himself. The DVLA defines alcohol misuse as 'a state that causes, because of consumption of alcohol, disturbance of behaviour, related disease or other consequences likely to cause the patient, their family or society present or future harm and that may or may not be associated with dependence'. Further UK information can be accessed at www.gov.uk/alcohol-problems-and-driving.

With regards to the above, A should fill out the DVLA's DR1 form, which will ask him pertinent questions about his alcohol history (29). Guidance for clinicians can be sought by accessing https://assets.publishing.service.gov.uk/government/uploads/system/uploads/attachment_data/file/670819/assessing-fitness-to-drive-a-guide-for-medical-professionals.pdf.

After submitting the completed form, the DVLA will request medical opinions from his clinicians on his fitness to drive and could request an independent assessment too. This usually takes around six weeks to determine whether the driving licence should be issued, refused or revoked. Licence holders normally retain entitlement to drive under Section 88 of the Road Traffic Act 1988. However, doctors in charge of the patient's care should advise the driver as to whether or not it is safe for them to continue driving during this pending period. Patients who ignore medical advice must be reminded that this may affect insurance cover and could ultimately lead to licence withdrawal.

For persistent alcohol misuse, group 1 (car and motorcycle) drivers will have their licence refused or revoked until at least six months of controlled drinking or abstinence. If an individual wishes to dispute a DVLA outcome, they can write to the DVLA and their local magistrates court but must do so within six months of this decision.

If A refused DVLA self-disclosure, the doctor must immediately notify DVLA on his behalf and should inform the patient of this action, although the latter is not compulsory. Disclosure involves filling out a DVLA medical notification and emailing it to medadviser@dvla.gsi.gov.uk (30). Any clinical advice given to A must be documented in his medical notes as this may be required for future medico-legal proceedings

Q 5) True

It could be argued that football's 'macho' culture creates an environment where excessive alcohol consumption is readily tolerated and accepted, a view supported by David Cotterill's professional playing experience. David is an ex-professional Welsh international footballer, who is a now a passionate ambassador for improving mental health and addiction support within football.

Historically, alcohol brands have successfully aligned themselves through lucrative football advertising and sponsorship deals. Of concern, gambling outlets are now replacing alcohol's dominance in sponsorship, another potential behavioural addiction.

During the mid-1990s, Arsene Wenger (ex-Arsenal club manager) was one of the first to develop an English football club culture that encouraged alcohol moderation. Another watershed moment was in 2011 when the Football Association collaborated with Time to Change, an educational mental health resource, to create the 'Footballers' Guidebook, Life as a Professional Footballer and How to Handle It'. This included material dedicated to alcohol misuse within the professional game. (The latest PFA guidance on wellbeing for players can be found at www.thepfa.com/wellbeing/mental-health-and-football.) Also, Fédération Internationale de Football Association, the international governing body of football, has created formal guidelines for players on alcohol consumption and its ergolytic effects (31).

Footballers who are part of England's PFA national network now have access to 24/7 telephone counselling and funding towards private behavioural addiction treatment. There are also several sporting bodies that visit clubs to provide educational seminars on addictions. These resources should become available to all professional footballer unions, so that former players can readily access support too. The English Football League's recent two-year sponsorship deal (2018/19–2019/20) with the mental health charity Mind© is a landmark step aiming to provide stigma-free mental health awareness within football.

Acknowledgements

Within harmful alcohol misuse and addiction support we recognise that there are different ways that mental health professionals may assess this disorder. This chapter merely provides a suggested consultation template and we accept that there may be variations to this format.

Summary of the Chapter and the Topics Covered

- How to investigate and manage alcohol-related disorders in football
- Risk factors and manifestations of alcohol misuse in the elite football setting
- Potential barriers for footballers wishing to seek treatment for alcohol misuse
- Challenges associated with retirement from professional football
- The role of confidentiality working as a sports clinician in elite sport
- How culture can impact on health-related behaviour within a sport

References

1. Prochaska JO, DiClemente CC, Norcross JC. In search of how people change: Applications to the addictive behaviors. *American Psychologist*. 1992; 47:1102–14.

2. Sullivan JT, Sykara K, Schneiderman J, Naranjo CA, Sellers EM. Assessment of alcohol withdrawal: The revised Clinical Institute Withdrawal Assessment for Alcohol Scale (CIWA-Ar). *Br J Addict*. 1989;84:1353–7.

3. World Health Organization. *AUDIT, the Alcohol Use Disorders Identification Test*. 1989;Document No.WHO/MNH/DAT/89.4.

4. Mayfield,D, McLeod G, Hall P. The CAGE Questionnaire: Validation of a new alcohol screening instrument. *Am J Psychiatry*. 1974;*131*(10):1121–3.

5. National Institute of Health and Care Excellence. *Alcohol-Use Disorders: Diagnosis, Assessment and Management of Harmful Drinking and Alcohol Dependence (CG115)*, 2011. Available from: www.nice.org.uk/guidance/cg115

6. Reardon CL, Hainline B, Aron CM, Baron D, Baum AL, Bindra A, et al. Mental health in elite athletes: International Olympic Committee consensus statement (2019). *Br J Sports Med*. 2019;53 (11):667–99. Available from: www.ncbi.nlm.nih.gov/pubmed/31097450

7. Hainline B, Reardon CL. Breaking a taboo: Why the International Olympic Committee convened experts to develop a consensus statement on mental health in elite athletes. *Br J Sports Med*. 2019;0:1–4. doi:10.1136/bjsports-2019-100681

8. Castaldelli-Maia JM, Gallinaro JGM, Falcão RC, Gouttebarge V, Hitchcock ME, Hainline B, et al. Mental health symptoms and disorders in elite athletes: A systematic review on cultural influencers and barriers to athletes seeking treatment. *Br J Sports Med*. 2019; 53:707–721. doi:10.1136/bjsports-2019-100710

9. DiClemente CC, Bellino LE, Neavins TM. Motivation for change and alcohol treatment. *Alcohol Research & Health*. 1999; 23;2: 86–92.

10. Edwards AG, Rollnick S. Outcome studies of brief alcohol intervention in general practice: The problem of lost subjects. *Addiction.* 1997; 92(12):1699–704.

11. Miller WR, Rollnick S. *Motivational Interviewing: Preparing People for Change.* 2nd edition. New York, Guilford, 2002.

12. American Psychiatric Association. *Practice Guideline for the Treatment of Patients with Substance Misuse Disorders.* Work group on substance use disorders, 2nd edition. 2010.

13. Walters P, Hearn A, Currie A. Substance misuse. In, Currie A and Owen B, *Sport Psychiatry.* Oxford Psychiatry Library, 2016.

14. Lingford-Hughes AR, Welch S, Peters L, Nutt DJ. BAP updated guidelines: evidence-based guidelines for the pharmacological management of substance abuse, harmful use, addiction and comorbidity: Recommendations from BAP. *J Psychopharmacol.* 2012; 26(7):899–952.

15. Mason BJ, Goodman AM, Chabac S, Lehert P. Effect of oral acamprosate on abstinence in patients with alcohol dependence in a double-blind, placebo-controlled trial: The role of patient motivation. *J Psychiatr Res.* 2006;40:383–93.

16. Semple D, Smyth R. *Oxford Handbook of Psychiatry.* London: Oxford University Press. 2013.

17. BMJ Best Practice. *Alcohol-Use Disorders.* 2018. Available from: http://bestpractice.bmj.com/topics/en-us/198

18. Engleman E, Rodd ZA, Bell RL, et al. The role of 5-HT3 receptors in drug abuse and as a target for pharmacotherapy. *CNS Neurol Disord Drug Targets.* 2008; 7(5):454–67.

19. Green GA, Uryasz FD, Petr TA, et al. NCAA study of substance use and abuse habits of college student-athletes. *Clin J Sport Med.* 2001;11:51–6.

20. Gouttebarge V, Aoki H, Kerkhoffs G. Symptoms of common mental disorders and adverse health behaviours in male professional soccer players. *J Hum Kinet.* 2015;49:277–86.

21. McDuff D, Stull T, Castaldelli-Maia JM, Hitchcock ME, Hainline B, Reardon CL. Recreational and ergogenic substance use and substance use disorders in elite athletes: A narrative review. *Br J Sports Med.* 2019;0:1–7.

22. Gouttebarge V, Frings-Dresen MHW, Sluiter JK. Mental and psychosocial health among current and former professional footballers. *Occupational Medicine.* 2015;65:190–6.

23. Gouttebarge V, Castaldelli-Maia JM, Gorczynski P, Hainline B, Hitchcock ME, Kerkhoffs GM, et al. Occurrence of mental health symptoms and disorders in current and former elite athletes: A systematic review and meta-analysis. *Br J Sports Med.* 2019;53:700–7.

24. Barnes MJ. Alcohol: Impact on sports performance and recovery in male athletes. *Sports Med.* 2014;44:909–19.

25. Morgan MY, Ritson B. *Alcohol and Health.* London. Medical Council on Alcoholism.1998.

26. Taylor D, Barnes TRE, Young AH. Addictions and substance misuse. *The Maudsley Prescribing Guidelines,* 13th edition. Wiley-Blackwell. 2018.

27. Holvey C and Torrens N. *Guy's and St Thomas' Clinical Guidelines DTC Reference 10052a.* 2010.

28. Waddington I, Roderick M. Management of medical confidentiality in English professional football clubs: Some ethical problems and issues. *Br J Sports Med.* 2002;36:118–23.

29. DVLA Report your medical condition (Form DR1). Available from: www.gov.uk/government/publications/dr1-online-confidential-medical-information

30. DVLA Notification form for healthcare professionals. Available from: https://assets.publishing.service.gov.uk/government/upl oads/system/uploads/attachment_data/file/506349/DOM3854_230216.pdf

31. FIFA Medical Assessment and Research Centre. *Nutrition for Football; A practical guide for eating and drinking for health and performance,* 2010. Available from: www.fifa.com/mm/document/footballdevelop ment/medical51/55/15/ nutritionbooklet_neue2010.pdf

Golf: Alcohol, Anxiety and Sleep Problems

Shane Creado, Phil Hopley and Andrew Murray
Athlete expert advisor: Marsha Hull

Within sports psychiatry it is well recognised that recreational golf participation can be beneficial for physical health and wellbeing (1). Professional golfers similar to the general population can experience work-related stress, relationship challenges, financial pressures and loneliness (2). This may be linked with pro golfers spending an average 30 weeks/year away from their family homes with their support teams. This high frequency of travel makes continuity of psychological care challenging.

While a range of personalities play professional golf, common personality traits include tendencies towards perfectionism, introspection, introversion and self-criticism. Psychiatric disorders often seen in professional golfers include affective disorders, e.g. depression and anxiety, ADHD and obsessive compulsive disorder (OCD). Given the diverse demographic of golfers, not only should offered psychiatric treatment be evidence-based but it must respect the golfer's cultural background too.

Background

SR is a 50-year-old former professional golfer. Five years ago, he had a lower back injury which required extensive physiotherapy. He never fully recovered and subsequently retired from the professional golfers' tour. During this time, he had become increasingly worried about the future, about whether he could even play golf socially and became concerned about his financial security. S's sleep became disrupted and his alcohol consumption increased, drinking bourbon (whisky) most evenings. Also, he was going through divorce proceedings initiated by his wife, following frequent arguments and a breakdown in their marriage.

His best friend and former caddie became concerned about his mental health and encouraged him to seek professional mental health care. Eventually S had agreed to see a sports psychiatrist and a copy of the consultation notes are outlined below.

Presenting Complaint

'I am caught up in a spiral of worrying about the future, losing everything I loved and I have lost hope for a happy life. I cannot seem to get myself out of it. I feel tense, on edge and haven't had a good night's sleep in years.'

History of Presenting Complaint

Following his back injury he had been unable to play golf again and was taking strong medication that provided him with some pain relief and allowed him an acceptable range of movement. Since then, he confessed to experiencing a pattern of self-defeating thoughts, worries about whether he could ever play golf again, poor sleep, frequent disagreements with his wife and drinking larger amounts of alcohol. He justified the alcohol consumption as it helped him fall asleep and cope with his wife's recent initiation of divorce proceedings.

In terms of his back pain, towards the end of his golfing career he was initially diagnosed with lumbar spondylosis and associated radiculopathy, as well as a mild spondylolisthesis at L5–L6. After he had discussed the prognosis with several surgeons and his primary care physician, S opted for the conservative management route, with physical conditioning, physiotherapy and medication. His symptoms never improved and pain limited his movements. As a result, he was unable to play golf. He had constant pain, at a level of L5 on the Visual Analogue Scale, exacerbated (up to 9) by certain movements and shooting pains into the back of both legs. He discontinued physiotherapy several months ago, as he did not believe this had made any difference. He continued to take various analgesic medications. Medication adherence was variable as he believed these medications were contributing to his daytime tiredness.

Along with his back pain, S complained about his disrupted sleep pattern. He would often doze off watching TV on the couch, and if he tried to sleep in his bed, he would invariably start to worry and be unable to fall asleep. Most nights, he woke up around 2am, and then it would be a challenge for him to fall back asleep, worrying about the next day and how sleepy he would be. Variable things would wake him up in the middle of the night. Sometimes he would wake up gasping for air or be suffering from distressing nightmares about being chased. Of note, his wife had informed him that she had heard him snoring loudly 'like gasping', even though she was sleeping in an adjacent room with ear plugs in. He had put on considerable amounts of weight (15kg) over the past year. He drank approximately six cups of strong coffee throughout the day.

S got anything from 3 to 10 hours of sleep at night, not counting daytime naps. Most days, he woke in the late morning, feeling unrefreshed, with a dry mouth and a dull headache. He rarely felt well rested, and looked forward to his afternoon 'siesta' after lunch, when he found himself once again dozing on the couch for a couple of hours. S believed poor sleep was one of his major problems and if corrected would alleviate many of his other difficulties and help him to 'think straight'. He had tried various pharmacological approaches (zolpidem, melatonin and temazepam) over the years with little success, although he admitted to 'never giving them a proper go'. S had always had poor sleep in and around major golf competitions although this had now taken over his life.

He had never been medically evaluated for a potential sleeping disorder. When asked, S denied a history of restless leg syndrome (an uncomfortable sensation in the legs, worse at night, worse with periods of immobility and relieved with movement) and his wife denied any reports of him sleep talking, sleep walking or acting out his dreams at night.

Although he endorsed daytime sleepiness, this was in the context of his fragmented night time sleep. He denied symptoms that would be suspicious of a central nervous system hypersomnia (sleepiness despite adequate night time sleep, cataplexy, hypnagogic or hypnopompic hallucinations or sleep paralysis).

Due to S's preoccupation with his somatic complaints, he was encouraged to discuss his mental health concerns. S felt that he was always on edge and that his muscles were 'tight'. He anticipated 'bad news' every day and had begun to ignore phone calls from his divorce lawyer, in fear of what they may say. When anxiety built up, he described episodes of uncontrollable shaking, muscle tension, heavy sweating, fast breathing and 'getting stuck in one spot'. This was one of the main reasons he rarely went out and he was fearful of having a heart attack if he left the house. These symptoms occurred on most days, around four times daily, and it usually took 10 minutes for symptoms to dissipate. The symptoms were usually provoked by a thought. S recalled similar symptoms during his golfing career but nowhere close to the same intensity.

Regarding symptoms of depression, he reported low mood (rated today at 3/10), insomnia as described, although he enjoyed his hobbies when his energy levels and chronic pain permitted him to go fishing or see old friends. He denied suicidal ideation, intent, plans or means. On direct questioning there were no reported symptoms of mania, psychosis, OCD-type symptoms, ADHD- or PTSD-associated symptoms.

Past Psychiatric History

No previous psychiatric history was reported.

Family History

S was adopted aged six and never knew his biological parents. He did not have memories of childhood prior to adoption. He understood that his biological home environment was unstable with violence and drug misuse.

He had two younger biological siblings but had not stayed in close contact with either of them. He knew that his brother, aged 46, had a suspected drinking problem and sleep apnoea and that his 45-year-old sister suffered with anxiety and PTSD.

Past Medical History

Lumbar spondylosis and associated radiculopathy

Spondylolisthesis at L5–L6

Obesity (BMI 31)

Hypertension

Hypercholesterolemia

Medication

Paracetamol 1g four times daily (pain)

Pregabalin 100mg three times daily (radiculopathy)

Lisinopril 20mg once daily (hypertension)

Oxycodone HCL 10–20mg as required, maximum 40mg daily (back pain)

Zolpidem tartrate 10mg once at night (insomnia, not effective, intermittently compliant)

Social History

S was currently married, but in the midst of a divorce, initiated by his wife of 23 years. They still lived in the same home they shared, near Daytona Beach, Florida, but in separate rooms and living 'different lives'. She cooked her meals while he snacked on chocolate and crisps or ordered take-away food. He was currently working with a divorce lawyer, although was unsure whether he actually wanted a divorce, and was going along with this to respect his wife's wishes. He found it very difficult to address his feelings with regards to this and had given up hope of trying to salvage his marriage.

He rarely went out, unless a close friend dropped by his house and coaxed him to step outside for a walk and a 'catch up'. Apart from this, he had little socialisation. He used to be fond of playing the guitar, but had not played in over a year. He spent most of the day watching TV, eating and dozing periodically. He had a strong Christian faith, but had not attended a church service, apart from Easter and Christmas, in recent years. He did not have any children.

There were no reported financial concerns at present although this might change depending on the outcome of the divorce.

S's use of alcohol was as outlined above. He denied a history of complicated alcohol withdrawals (tremors, visual hallucinations, delirium tremens or seizures). On direct questioning there was no reported relief drinking, compulsion to drink or primacy of alcohol-seeking behaviour.

He also denied prior or current use or abuse of other recreational, illicit or prescription drugs.

Personal History

S did not know his birth history but suspected that he may have been exposed to illicit substances and alcohol in utero. He was adopted at age six and was raised in North Carolina, with his two younger siblings. All three of them went to private schools and his adopted parents provided a stable and comfortable home environment. His father was a successful lawyer and a member of prestigious golf clubs. He encouraged S to play golf from an early age.

At school he was bright and came in the top half of his class. However, he had a strong preference for sports and underachieved academically in his later school years as he devoted more time to playing golf. S said he focused on golf from as 'long ago as I can remember and nothing else mattered'. He had not played any other sports regularly. He won the club junior championship for three successive years aged 14–16 and the following year he won the full club championship aged 17. He was accepted into a renowned university to play golf on a full scholarship. S played in local, regional and national amateur tournaments in his late teens and early twenties with a reasonable degree of success given his age. He subsequently left university, turned professional and played regularly at an elite level.

S met his wife while playing amateur tournaments where she was working for a sports agency that managed golfers. She became his manager/agent and they would travel around on tour together.

Pre-Morbid Personality

S described himself as being serious, introspective, motivated and practical.

Forensic History

No history of any offending behaviour.

Collateral History

S's wife explained that they currently lived like room-mates, rather than partners. She could have moved out of the house, but because she was concerned about his mental state, she still lived in the same house. She elaborated that prior to initiating divorce proceedings she tried to get S to seek professional counselling, as she worried about his depression, which he seemed to numb with alcohol. He was adamant that he was not 'an alcoholic' and did not need any professional help. When her suggestions for him to get help were repeatedly rejected, she suggested couples' counselling, which he also dismissed and rejected. Growing up, she had seen her mother struggle in an abusive relationship with an alcoholic step-father, and she had promised herself at an early age to not let history repeat itself. Seeing what had happened to S had hurt her deeply, while feeling helpless to effect a positive change in his life. She tearfully recounted their early days, their hopes to start a business designing golf courses, to travel and have a family, all of which had abruptly ended. On careful reflection, she felt that everything in S's life revolved around his goals and desires, and she felt like an accessory in his world-view. She believed that S's complete disregard to engage in a healthy lifestyle and marriage had primarily led her to seek a divorce.

Mental State Examination

S presented as a 50-year-old obese Caucasian male. He was poorly kempt, wearing a cap, t-shirt with a few stains and was unshaven. He was pleasant in his interactions but demonstrated avoidant eye contact and was intermittently tearful. There was no evidence of psychomotor retardation and there was a normal speech pattern in rate, tone and volume. He initially appeared anxious although he did not demonstrate any acute alcohol with-drawal. His affect was restricted and mood was congruent, describing it as 'worried and irritated'. There was no evidence of disordered thought. His thought content did not demonstrate any evidence of delusions, obsessions, phobias or suicidal thoughts. He was fully orientated in time, place and person.

S possessed relatively good insight into his life situation, unhealthy habits, affective distress and the impact of his somatic complaints. He had partial insight into his increasing alcohol consumption. However, he was motivated to seek professional support including psychological support.

Risk Assessment

Self: There was no evidence of suicidal ideation or active suicidal or DSH plans. His current alcohol consumption potentially placed him at risk of sleep disruption, weight gain, mood disorders, cognitive impairment and other long-term physical health risks if not addressed. There was an increased risk for sleep apnoea, associated depression and anxiety.

Others: Nil identified.

Protective factors: S showed some motivation to address his unhealthy lifestyle, anxiety, depression and sleep disruptions and engage in professional support, and had some insight into the risks associated with his current trajectory.

Investigations

GAD-7 (for anxiety severity): 15

PHQ-9 (for depression severity): 19

STOP-Bang questionnaire (for sleep apnoea): Positive

Epworth Sleepiness Scale: 12

Blood tests: Full blood count, renal function, liver function (including GGT), thyroid function, vitamin D, hormone testing, random glucose and HbA1c, iron panel all within normal parameters.

Formulation

S presented as a 55-year-old former professional golfer who was experiencing prominent anxiety symptoms and disrupted sleep pattern with a significant impact on social functioning. Chronic pain had forced him to prematurely retire from his golfing career.

In terms of predisposing factors, S possessed sub-threshold symptoms of anxiety and sleep disturbance even during his active sporting career. There was a family history of both mood disorder and substance abuse.

His recent marital breakdown along with chronic back pain status were the most likely factors that had precipitated his current mental state. These were linked with sedentary behaviour, weight gain and increased alcohol use all of which are known to increase the risk of sleep apnoea, mood disorders and further sleep disruption. S demonstrated partial insight into his difficulties and appeared motivated to address his overall situation, particularly his sleep.

Plan

- S was given free access to an online mental health resource website and was referred to a local counselling service to help him address his current divorce situation. He agreed to ask his wife to see whether she would consider attending couples' therapy with him
- S was referred to a psychologist with a view to individual CBT to address anxiety symptoms
- He was provided with information about a local alcohol peer-support group meeting that he would be welcome to attend
- S was referred to a community physiotherapist to help address his back pain and promote safe, moderate-intensity physical activity
- S was provided with a sleep hygiene booklet which advised him to:
  - Take regular sleep hours
  - Maintain a sleep and mood diary
  - Create a restful sleep environment
  - Engage in moderate levels of physical activity (back injury permitting)
  - Replace caffeinated drinks in the evening with herbal or decaffeinated teas

○ Download a free mobile app to help him utilise relaxation and breathing techniques prior to bedtime

○ Avoid visual stimulation (TV, laptops, mobile phone screen time) one to two hours prior to sleep

- His primary care physician was given advice on potential anxiolytic medication options that could be offered
- S was offered a psychiatric outpatient follow up appointment in six weeks' time to review his mental state and response to the current treatment care plan

Questions

Q 1 Based on the case history, which of the following diagnoses should be included in the initial differential diagnosis?
A. GAD
B. Alcohol dependence syndrome
C. Harmful use of alcohol
D. PTSD
E. MDD

Q 2 Which of the following are essential further investigations in S's case to ensure the treatment plan is optimised?
A. Collateral history
B. Urine drug screen
C. MRI brain scan
D. DNA testing for psycho-pharmacogenetic profile
E. Full physical examination

Q 3 Assuming a primary diagnosis of GAD and a secondary diagnosis of harmful use of alcohol, which of the following should always be included in an initial treatment plan?
A. Anti-anxiety medication
B. Advice on lifestyle factors
C. Referral for individual psychological therapy
D. Advice on self-help strategies
E. Referral for group therapy support

Q 4 Which of the following statements are correct regarding anxiety disorders?
A. Catastrophic thinking is common to several anxiety disorders
B. PTSD develops within weeks of the priming traumatic event
C. Pharmacological treatment should be the first-line option for GAD
D. Anxiety disorders can commonly mimic medical conditions leading to incorrect self-diagnosis and worsening of symptoms
E. All of the above statements are correct

Q 5 Based on the case history, which of the following sleep disorders should be included in the initial differential diagnosis?
   A. Chronic insomnia disorder
   B. Short-term insomnia disorder
   C. Insomnia due to alcohol consumption
   D. Sleep apnoea
   E. All of the above

Answers

Q 1) A, C, E

The core presenting feature for S is that of anxiety. S developed understandable worries regarding his health and career in response to a career-ending injury. His livelihood along with his physical health had been affected. In the early stages this would be regarded as a psychological reaction best termed an 'adjustment disorder' (International Classification of Diseases ICD-10 code: F43.2).

In ICD-10 GAD (F41.1) requires the presence of marked excessive worry or fear lasting six months or longer (3). Associated symptoms include fatigue, reduced concentration, irritability, sleep disturbance, restlessness, muscle tension and associated physiological symptoms (tachycardia, chest tension, shortness of breath, sweating, dizziness, etc.). Ruminating is common in both anxiety and depression and results in repetitively going over a thought or a problem without completion. There is considerable overlap between anxiety disorders and mood disorders in the context of medical treatment options.

MDD (ICD-10 code: F32) should also be considered in this case as S presented with low mood, loss of pleasure, irritability, sleep disturbance, reduced concentration and lowered energy. Other key depressive symptoms are not evident: loss of appetite, weight loss, early morning wakening, diurnal mood variation, marked hopelessness and suicidal thoughts.

Within the history, S demonstrated a clear increase in the use of alcohol to above recommended limits. This was initially as a means of self-medicating initial insomnia, in keeping with harmful use of alcohol (ICD-10 code: F10.1) (4). This often presents as a co-morbidity with psychiatric illness. The case history has outlined one or two indicators of alcohol dependence syndrome: narrowing of the repertoire of drinking and (probably) increased tolerance. There is no evidence of withdrawal symptoms, primacy of alcohol seeking, compulsion to drink, relief drinking for withdrawal or rapid re-instatement after a period of abstinence. Therefore, the criteria for alcohol dependence syndrome (ICD-10 code F10.2) has not been met. However, clinicians should always bear in mind the possibility of patient minimisation driven by denial as a reason for inaccuracy in the information obtained at an initial assessment.

S did not present with any evidence of PTSD (ICD-10 code: F43.1) such as intrusive recollections of a traumatic incident (as flashbacks or nightmares), autonomic hyperarousal and avoidance of reminders or triggers of the original trauma. Symptoms of PTSD typically arise within three months of a major trauma and last for not less than one month. Similar reactions of a shorter duration are most likely to be due to an acute stress reaction (ICD-10 code: F43.0).

Q 2) A, B, E

Psychiatric evaluations are subject to bias if they are solely based on the account of one individual. In this case, S was refusing consent to speak to the closest observant (his wife) due to concerns about the impact of his evaluation on the forthcoming divorce proceedings. Although it was unlikely that he would be willing to change his consent position, good practice would encourage the patient to speak to his lawyers and take advice on this point. The couple had no children and often fears of the psychiatric history being used as grounds in custody battles apply. In this case, this issue would not apply. Other reliable sources of collateral history could include his former caddy and any other close friends. Further sources of important information include his medical records.

All mental health presentations need to exclude organic causes or substance misuse that could explain the changes in mental state. A full physical examination is important at the initial consultation (5). S's history of alcohol misuse and the prescription of opiate analgesia mean that a screen for illicit/recreational drug misuse is important . However, in the absence of a history of head injury, seizures or objective cognitive impairment, an MRI brain scan is not essential.

Pharmacogenomic testing has become a fast-growing area within medicine including in psychiatric practice (6). Testing provides a DNA profile indicating an individual's gene profile for neurotransmitter receptors and CYP-450 enzymes. These are said to give predictive value to medication choice for all psychotropics by anticipating poor responders and fast/slow drug metabolisers. Although a valuable addition to the tools available to psychiatrists, this level of investigation is not regarded as essential at this stage.

Q 3) B, C, D

The first-line treatment of anxiety disorders should be evidence-based psychological interventions (7). These are recommended in preference to pharmacological treatment. The treatment of choice for GAD is CBT. However, while group therapy based on CBT lines may have a role to play it would not be regarded as a first-line intervention.

CBT helps the patient to understand different ways of thinking, behaving and reacting to situations that reduce anxiety and worry. Therapy can last anywhere between 10 and 20 sessions, with most people reporting significant symptom reduction after 10 sessions. CBT for GAD typically includes several of the following components:

○ **Relaxation training** to counter the physiological tendency for individuals to feel tense
○ **Cognitive restructuring** to focus on negative predictions about the future, and unhelpful attitudes about one's ability to cope with difficult situations
○ **Mindfulness** to practise bringing one's attention to the present moment in order to reduce rumination
○ **Systematic exposure** to help people face their fears and test their catastrophic predictions
○ **Problem-solving** to learn skills to effectively manage stress

Self-help is a key aspect to improving many if not all mental health conditions and patients can be empowered to take a pro-active role in their recovery. Many of the changes needed in order to manage anxiety can be addressed with self-help: diet/exercise/sleep hygiene/healthy alcohol consumption. In addition, access to good mental health online tools and apps has been made more readily available within the general population. This could allow lower-level and sub-threshold symptoms to be addressed in a less formal way.

If pharmacological options were to be considered for S's anxiety, it should be noted that he is already taking a recognised anti-anxiety drug, pregabalin, at a relatively high dose. One medication option would be to increase the dose to the recommended daily maximum of 600mg in divided doses.

The first-line medication option for GAD remains SSRI antidepressant medications (8). These include fluoxetine, citalopram, escitalopram, sertraline, paroxetine and vortioxetine. An explanation of the risk of short-term increase in anxiety and agitation is essential for patients starting SSRIs, and effective safety plans with follow up should be made in order to minimise any potential side effects.

Alternative options include duloxetine, an SNRI (selective serotonin and noradrenaline reuptake inhibitor) that is reported to provide relief for individuals suffering neuropathic pain (8). Some psychiatrists may offer duloxetine as a first line over an SSRI. Less commonly, low dose antipsychotics (e.g. olanzapine or quetiapine) can be used in the management of over-whelming anxiety. However, given S's recent weight gain and sedentary behaviour, there should be a high threshold before resorting to these options as both are associated with weight gain. More practical support options would include a review of his lifestyle factors.

S is no longer receiving the benefits inherent in regular exercise and social contact through meaningful activity. His diet is poor. His weight gain will most likely be impacting his sleep quality (apnoea) and his self-esteem. His harmful alcohol use will be interfering with sleep, exacerbating anxiety, lowering his mood and contributing to his weight gain. His alcohol use may also be reducing the effectiveness of his pregabalin. These combined factors have created a negative spiral of unhealthy behaviours/dysfunctional coping strategies.

Following simple psycho-education (explanation of the negative impact of these factors and the benefits of making change), attempts should be made to engage S in goal setting around small but sustainable changes in diet and alcohol consumption. Also, supporting S with the idea of reconnecting with friends and former colleagues and/or finding manage-able meaningful activity (e.g. researching non-physical work opportunities) may encourage him to explore these aspects of behavioural activation with a trained therapist.

Q 4)   A, B and D

Anxiety disorders have excessive worry as a core symptom. One type of such distorted thinking is catastrophising or anticipating the worst possible outcome/worst-case scenario (9). Catastrophising, however, is not pathognomonic for anxiety disorders as it is a common (possibly the commonest) form of cognitive distortion arising in anyone with or without mental health problems.

Catastrophising is best addressed through cognitive restructuring using a simple process called Check/Challenge/Change where the feared disastrous outcome is challenged by an analysis of the facts of the situation, i.e. 'when you thought this would happen, what actually happened?' This form of challenge allows the patient to possess less rigid/automatic cognitive responses to difficult events or unhelpful thoughts.

As previously outlined, NICE guidelines consider psychological therapy to be a first-line treatment intervention for anxiety (3). Anxiety disorders have a physiological element through autonomic stimulation. In extreme cases of panic disorder, sufferers fear that they are having a heart attack (palpitations and chest tightness) or a stroke (fainting, tension headaches). In such cases and in other types of anxiety disorders these physical symptoms may be misinterpreted and mistaken for acute medical conditions leading people to seek medical advice.

Physicians should be alert to these presentations but equally understand that medical and psychological co-morbidity are not uncommon. This is particularly important for patients with somatoform disorders (formerly called hypochondriasis) who repeatedly present with medically unexplained symptoms although may one day present with a genuine medical condition or emergency.

Q 5)   A and D

The International Classifications of Sleep Disorders, third edition (ICSD-3), has discarded the old diagnostic categories of primary and secondary insomnia. This was based on evidence demonstrating conclusively that specific factors contributing to insomnia are co-morbid, rather than causal. The diagnosis of insomnia is a clinical one and not based on laboratory or other investigations. For a diagnosis of chronic insomnia, the sleep disturbance and associated daytime symptoms should have been present for at least three months. Short-term insomnia disorder involves sleep disturbance and associated daytime sleepiness for less than three months (10) and S could not be diagnosed with this in view of the longer duration of his symptoms.

Other features of chronic or short-term insomnia include:

○ The reported sleep/wake complaints cannot be explained purely by inadequate opportunity or inadequate circumstances for sleep
○ The sleep disturbance and associated daytime symptoms occur at least three times per week
○ The sleep/wake difficulty is not better explained by another sleep disorder
○ One or more is reported: difficulty initiating sleep, difficulty maintaining sleep, waking up earlier than desired, resistance to going to bed on appropriate schedule, difficulty sleeping without parent or caregiver intervention
○ One or more of the following, related to the night time sleep difficulty: fatigue/malaise, attention/concentration/memory impairment, impaired social/family/occupational/academic performance, mood disturbance/irritability, daytime sleepiness, behavioural problems (hyperactivity, impulsivity, aggression), reduced motivation/energy/initiative, proneness for errors/accidents, concerns about or dissatisfaction with sleep (11)

In the case of S, we can assume that certain subtypes may apply to his insomnia, such as: inadequate sleep hygiene, insomnia due to mental disorder, insomnia due to medical condition (pain), insomnia due to alcohol (middle insomnia).

Alcohol may contribute to his sleep disturbance although a causal relationship cannot be confirmed, particularly as there are many contributing factors to S's condition. Additionally, 'insomnia due to alcohol consumption' is not a formal diagnostic label.

S presented with symptoms compatible with sleep apnoea, although this case study is focused on obstructive sleep apnoea (OSA). Approximately 3–7% of men and 2–5% of women have sleep apnoea (12). Some suggest that the prevalence may be much higher but since clinicians do not screen patients, OSA is often missed and may manifest as a complex syndrome in one of the conditions it is associated with, or contributes to. OSA is characterised by repetitive episodes of partial (hypopnoea) or complete (apnoea) upper airway obstruction *occurring during sleep*. By definition, apnoeic and hypopnoiec events last a minimum of 10 seconds (13). Sleep apnoea is associated with, and contributes to, type 2 diabetes, hypertension, pulmonary hypertension, cor pulmonale, gastro-oesophageal reflux disease, stroke, myocardial infarction, sudden death, heart failure and irregular heart rhythms. There is some evidence that suggests an overlap between the presence of sleep apnoea and MDD. Many people who are misdiagnosed with ADHD may in fact have undiagnosed sleep apnoea (14). Recent studies have indicated that sleep apnoea may be an independent risk factor for cancer and dementia.

Symptoms may include daytime sleepiness, non-restorative sleep, fatigue/insomnia symptoms and night time awakenings (with breath holding, gasping or choking). A bed partner may report issues such as snoring or breathing interruptions/pauses as evidenced in S's presentation(15).

A useful screening tool for OSA is the STOP-Bang questionnaire. This reviews potential OSA symptoms and indicates whether an individual is low ('Yes' to 0–2 questions), intermediate ('Yes' to 3–4 questions) or high risk ('Yes' to 5–8 questions) for this condition. If the answers to more than three questions come back 'Yes', with a certain degree of clinical suspicion, it would warrant a referral for a polysomnogram or a home sleep study. Based on the results of the testing, a sleep clinician may decide on auto positive airway pressure (PAP), a positional device, a mandibular advancement device, modification of lifestyle contributors (allergens, alcohol, medications like benzodiazepines) and weight loss or some combination of these. An in-lab PAP study is useful to determine the best pressures, and the type of device to use.

The details of sleep study findings such as apnoea-hypopnoea index (AHI), oximetry and treatment protocols are beyond the scope of this psychiatric chapter.

Summary of the Chapter and the Topics Covered

- How psychosocial stressors and mental illness can present in retired athletes
- Initial screen history of sleep disorders and management of insomnia
- Presence and diagnostic challenges of mental and physical health co-morbidity in athletes
- The assessment of GAD
- Biopsychosocial treatment options for anxiety disorders

References

1. Murray AD, Daines L, Archibald D, et al. The relationships between golf and health: A scoping review. *Br J of Sports Med.* 2017;51:12–19.

2. Fry J, Bloyce D. Life in the travelling circus: A study of loneliness, work stress, and money issues in touring professional golf. *Sociology of Sport Journal.* 2017;34 (2):148–59.

3. National Institute for Health and Care Excellence. *Generalised Anxiety Disorder and Panic Disorder in Adults: Management Clinical Guideline* (CG-113). Updated July 2019. 2011.

4. World Health Organization. *The ICD-10 Classification of Mental and Behavioural Disorders: Clinical Descriptions and Diagnostic Guidelines.* Geneva. World Health Organization. 1992.

5. Bystritsky A, Khalsa SS, Cameron ME, Schiffman J. Current diagnosis and treatment of anxiety disorders. *Pharmacy and Therapeutics (P & T).*2013;38 (1):30–57.

6. Kitzmiller JP, Groen DK, Phelps MA, Sadee W. Pharmacogenomic testing: Relevance in medical practice: why drugs work in some patients but not in others. *Cleve Clin J Med.* 2011; 78(4):243–57.

7. Hunot V, Churchill R, Teixeira V, Silva de Lima M. Psychological therapies for generalised anxiety disorder. *Cochrane Database of Systematic Reviews.* 2007;(1).

8. Farach FJ, Pruitt LD, Jun JJ, Jerud AB, Zoellner L, Roy-Byrne PP. Pharmacological treatment of anxiety disorders: Current treatments and future directions. *Journal of Anxiety Disorders.* (2012);26(8):833–43.

9. Grohol, J. *What is Catastrophizing?* Psych Central article. https://psychcentral.com/lib/what-is-catastrophizing. 2018.

10. J. Edinger, D. Buysse, K. Lichstein, et al. *Insomnia, Short-Term Insomnia Disorder. International Classification of Sleep Disorders,* 3rd edition. American Academy of Sleep Medicine. 2014; p. 21–42.

11. Edinger J, Buysse DK, Lichstein K, et al. *Insomnia, Chronic Insomnia Disorder. International Classification of Sleep Disorders,* 3rd edition. American Academy of Sleep Medicine. 2014; p. 21–22.

12. Berry R, Lee-Chiong T, Marcus C, et al. *Sleep Related Breathing Disorders, Obstructive Sleep Apnoea Disorders. International Classification of Sleep Disorders,* 3rd edition. American Academy of Sleep Medicine. 2014; p. 55–56.

13. Berry R, Lee-Chiong T, Marcus C, et al. *Sleep Related Breathing Disorders, Obstructive Sleep Apnoea Disorders. International Classification of Sleep Disorders,* 3rd edition. American Academy of Sleep Medicine. 2014; p. 54.

14. Berry R, Lee-Chiong T, Marcus C, et al. *Sleep Related Breathing Disorders, Obstructive Sleep Apnoea Disorders. International Classification of Sleep Disorders,* 3rd edition. American Academy of Sleep Medicine. 2014; p. 55.

15. Berry R, Lee-Chiong T, Marcus C, et al. *Sleep Related Breathing Disorders, Obstructive Sleep Apnoea Disorders. International Classification of Sleep Disorders,* 3rd edition. American Academy of Sleep Medicine. 2014; p. 53.

Rugby: Concussion and Mental Health Symptoms

Thomas McCabe, Catherine Lester and Simon Kemp

Athlete expert advisor: Rob Vickerman

Physical health concerns and injuries can be a difficult time for athletes. Psychological distress and uncertainty with regards to future sporting careers can emerge and symptoms of worry, anxiety distress and low mood may even reach clinical levels. Sports psychiatrists play an important role in the identification and management of these issues alongside the rest of the medical and support team.

Protocols around concussion and RTP (return to play) are improving but are not yet standardised across all sports settings although rugby union would be seen as taking a lead in the management of acute head injury. There is an emphasis on measuring cognitive functioning when considering the acute effects of a head impact and other mental health issues may take longer to manifest. In some cases they may not be identified at all or be 'overshadowed' by the primary presentation unless they are looked for specifically.

Background

BD is a 34-year-old semi-professional rugby union player and a part-time schoolteacher. Three years ago she suffered three concussions during one season and required a prolonged period of rest. Following an extended RTP (return to play) protocol, which involved a month away from any rugby contact and a gradual increase in physical activity, she was integrated back into the team environment although she always thought she never reached her previous level of performance.

B recently suffered another concussion in training. In the four months since then, she complained of headaches. These were difficult to treat and she voluntarily stood down from selection. She felt pressured by her coach to 'just get on with it' and to get back playing as soon as possible as the best way to deal with her symptoms. He had been unsympathetic to her concerns about a further head injury and had largely ignored her when around the club and team environment as a result. She planned to retire from rugby as, in addition to being unavailable as a result of injury, her present contract runs out at the end of the season in two months time.

She presented to her primary care physician with low mood. She was offered but declined a referral for CBT, due to its limited therapeutic effects in the past. Her primary care physician decided to refer her to a psychiatrist in the local community mental health team (CMHT) who had a special interest in sports psychiatry.

Presenting Complaint

'I've been feeling terrible recently, my mood is low and I can't see how my headaches are going to get better.'

History of Presenting Complaint

B had been suffering from low mood (which she rated as 2/10) for the past six months. She described feeling 'glum' most days and 'puts on a smile' when in company. Her husband had started to notice this and initially told her to 'snap out of it'. With time, he had realised this had made things worse. She believed he had become more understanding recently as she had tried to make plans for the future and he had seen her 'making more of an effort'. Without having the usual contact with her rugby team, she felt isolated and unable to 'get myself going again'.

She admitted experiencing a loss of interest in rugby – which she had seen as her 'life and the thing that has got me out of bed most mornings'. B was unclear of the precise chronology of her symptoms and specifically which came first – the last head injury or the deterioration in her mood. She thought that both issues were related. She admitted to decreased motivation for any weight training or cardio fitness work and had subsequently gained weight.

Her concentration on everyday tasks such as prolonged conversation or reading had reduced. She had noticed this before with previous concussions. In addition, this time she felt tearful at even minor non-threatening stimuli, for example, a sad storyline in a television programme. She had been coping with work but felt exhausted at the end of the day and reported dozing on the couch in the evenings. She worried that work will be the next area of her life to suffer.

B also described increased anxiety around crowds of people and had avoided socialising with friends although she continued to go on walks with her husband and to do the weekly food shopping. She had been helping out with coaching the under-10s team at a nearby school and found this provided her with some solace. She enjoyed this because it 'brings me back to my younger days and I forget my problems'.

B described a poor sleep pattern that she said was 'broken throughout the night' and was wakening in the early hours of the morning. She blamed this on a chronic headache although admitted that her thoughts and worries had also contributed to this. B last slept well approximately six months ago, around the time of the most recent head injury. She reported a loss of libido and also that her temper with her husband had become much shorter. She was reluctant to discuss her home life in any further depth. She was hopeful for the future and wanted to throw herself into teaching.

Her rugby coach had made comments about her weight that had caused her great distress and left her feeling increasingly self-conscious. He had also spoken negatively about B to other members of the team when they had been training and had ignored her around the team environment. She felt powerless to address this and resented the coach as a result. Their relationship was good until recently but had now broken down and she had been afraid to speak to him about her plans to retire. B felt there was no way back into the first team as a result of both the conflict with coach and her loss of form and fitness. She felt she was losing her identity as a rugby player.

Past Psychiatric History

B had no significant past psychiatric history and had never seen a psychiatrist before. She completed an online CBT module following previous concussions but did not find it helpful.

She had experienced three head injury events in an eight-month period, three seasons ago. The most serious involved head contact with the ground after fielding a high ball and falling from a height. There was loss of consciousness and she required neck stabilisation and an overnight stay in hospital. Following this she had a week off work due to fatigue and nausea, which subsided with rest. Following the standard enhanced care graduated RTP pathway she played in a match a week after that. Shortly after this she received a blow to the side of the head from a knee during a tackle in a match. She was not removed from the field of play at the time of the collision but described 'brain fog' and a headache after the game. B specified that this was when she started to feel more 'on edge' and her on-field performance suffered as result. She never regained the confidence to 'get up in the air' to take high balls, and moved from her inside centre position on to the wing to avoid heavy tackling. B had developed more kicking strategies in her attack to avoid contacts and wondered whether this was also related to loss of confidence. She took advice from her team physiotherapist and did not play for three months. She continued with light aerobic fitness during this time but without instruction from medical personnel nor a structured RTP plan. She discussed her problems with a primary care physician who deemed her safe for RTP after three months.

Family History

There was no significant family history of mental illness or forensic history. Specifically there was no history of dementia, neurocognitive disorder, addictions or other major mental health illness within the immediate family.

Past Medical History

She was awaiting a neurology outpatient appointment for chronic headache on the background of her head injury. This followed a referral made by her primary care physician

Traumatic fracture of right 5th metatarsal (four years ago)

Right knee medial collateral injury – conservative management (seven years ago)

Medication

Regular Paracetamol 1g QDS

Ibuprofen 400mg TDS

Codeine 60mg as required for headache – using approximately once weekly

Social History

B lives with her husband within their own home. They intended to start a family once her rugby playing career was over.

She reported binge alcohol drinking at team bonding sessions where new players are initiated into the team and players pay for any factitious 'fines' for offences throughout the season by drinking large amounts of alcohol or accepting a degrading 'challenge'. These sessions are held around six times in a season. Otherwise she had one large glass of red wine on a Friday evening with food. She denied any recreational drug use.

Personal History

She was born and raised in a northern England town and was unaware of any childhood developmental delays. She was popular among her peers and from an early age played regular rugby for her local boys' team. She first played adult women's rugby at 18.

Her parents were farmers, in a happy relationship and supportive of her academically and in sporting pursuits. She played several sports in her youth including rugby, netball, athletics and horse riding. She has one younger brother who also plays rugby as a professional. She has a close relationship with all her family. They are concerned about her and have seen an obvious difference in her but do not know the reason why.

B was educated at a local state school. She achieved three Cs at A-level and went to university where she graduated with a degree in teaching. After university she played semi-professionally at a premiership team while also working as a primary school teacher. She has stayed with the same club throughout her career. She has played 14 times for the national team in the autumn internationals although not within the last four years. She has not been selected for a world cup campaign or been seen as a regular starter for the national team. B blamed this on never being 'big enough' and relying instead on pace and footwork to avoid contact. She was voted 'player of the year' for three years running for her club. She played mainly at inside centre or wing and had worn a scrum cap all of her career.

Her head teacher had been largely supportive of her in recent years. She was managing work well and was hopeful of applying for a full-time job within the same school in the next 12 months when she retired from professional rugby.

She met her husband of six years after leaving university. He is a similar age and works as an accountant.

Pre-Morbid Personality

B described herself as previously hard-working and committed. Lacking motivation or drive was uncharacteristic of her. She was a sociable and family-orientated person. Her husband described her as outgoing, engaging and a lot of fun to be around.

Forensic History

There was no forensic history.

Collateral History

Her husband had been worried about her. He described her becoming withdrawn and occasionally irritable around the house.

Mental State Examination

B was dressed in her club tracksuit and clean trainers. She was well-kempt with long dark hair that was tied up in a bun. She had a lean and muscular physique. She was wearing earrings, her engagement and wedding rings, painted finger nails and subtle make up. She was pleasant and cooperative throughout the majority of assessment, although became irritable and slightly anxious towards the end when discussing treat-ment options. Her eye contact was intense at times. There were no obvious speech abnormalities and her speech was normal in rhythm, rate and tone. She did not appear to be in pain nor to have any ongoing manifestations of headache. She did not seem as forthcoming with her thoughts and feelings when her husband was present. Her mood was subjectively low (2/10) although objectively euthymic. There were no thoughts of harm to herself or others. There was no evidence of delusional thought content or perceptual abnormalities and specifically no hallucinations in any modality. Her basic cognition appeared intact with a MMSE score of 30/30. Her focus was on the previous head injury as the main cause for her current symptoms and problems. After discussion she was in more agreement with the medical complexity of her presentation and the uncertainty with regards to how much the previous head injury had impacted on her current symptoms. When presented with the diagnosis, she seemed to understand and was motivated to take ownership of her recovery.

There were no focal neurological signs on basic examination.

Risk Assessment

Self: there were no thoughts or plans of self-harm and no previous episodes of self-harm acts. Although less motivated in general she was able to maintain a good diet and adequate self-care. There was no unexplained loss of consciousness or seizure-like activity.

Others: although a little more irritable this posed no risk to others and there was no history of any physical violence or use of weapons.

Protective factors: her family and friends were aware of her difficulties and supportive. She was aware of which emergency mental health services were available and willing to use them should things get worse.

Investigations

No recent blood tests had been taken.

A standard MRI head scan was performed two months previously because of prolonged headaches. It was unremarkable, with no evidence of any changes and in particular no cerebral atrophy, space-occupying lesion, cranial fracture, intracranial bleed or subdural haematoma.

Case Formulation

B presented as a 34-year-old rugby player with a depressive episode on a background of head trauma and impending retirement from sport. There had been a significant effect on her functioning at home and within the team environment, to the extent that she had planned her career transition after rugby. She had been in supportive sporting and family environments for the majority of her life but the security she previously experienced within sport had changed and she now felt unsupported by her coach. This had additionally impacted on her decision to transition out of sport.

She has had several head injuries, both historical and recent and each without regular or close medical supervision. She had received little advice or guidance in relation to management either of the current injury or with short- to medium-term rugby career plans. These factors along with her perceived loss of form had led her to plan her retirement, which, despite her emotional frailty, she had proactively addressed.

Plan

- B was offered a further course of CBT with a trained therapist. She considered this but eventually declined. She was given information on free online CBT-based resources and mobile apps

- She agreed to an antidepressant medication trial of fluoxetine 20mg OD (an SSRI). Her primary care physician had been requested to monitor her medication tolerance and agreed to review her mental state in two weeks' time
- She agreed to provisionally defer a final decision on retirement in the expectation that an appropriate treatment plan would improve her symptoms
- An outpatient psychiatric review with the same psychiatrist was arranged in four weeks' time to assess progress, medication side effects, risk and medication dose

Questions

Q 1 What is the primary diagnosis?
   A. MDD
   B. Adjustment disorder
   C. Persistent post-concussive symptoms
   D Anxiety disorder
   E. No formal mental health diagnosis

Q 2 Which of the following statements related to head injury management in sport are true?
   A. The strongest predictors for prolonged recovery following uncomplicated head trauma in sport are previous concussive injury and loss of consciousness
   B. Headache is the most common symptom of concussion 24 hours post injury
   C. Rule changes are being trialled in elite-level rugby in an attempt to reduce concussion incidence
   D. Mouth guards and scrum caps reduce the risk of concussion
   E. Injuries to other parts of the body (i.e. upper limb) have been shown to have a higher risk ratio following a diagnosed concussion rather than a non-concussive injury

Q 3 Which of the following statements regarding retirement from sport are true?
   A. Guidance exists to assist players making decisions around retirement
   B. Epidemiological data suggest that retirement is a significant risk factor for mental health symptoms and disorders
   C. There is a difference in mental health outcomes between elite athletes forced to retire from sport and those taking voluntary retirement
   D. There is a significant association with forced retirement from rugby and alcohol misuse in later years
   E. Research informs us that the most common reason for early retirement in rugby is due to persisting neurocognitive symptoms

Q 4 Which of the following figures estimates the prevalence of depressive symptoms in professional rugby players?
   A. 5%
   B. 15%
   C. 28%
   D 42%
   E. 82%

Q 5 It is the club's sole responsibility to identify player or referee abuse and take appropriate action. True or False?

Answers

Q 1) A

The diagnosis is challenging and **four** of the above could reasonably apply. As has been seen in overtraining syndrome in athletes (1), there are times when the diagnosis is influenced by which professional the player presents to and the focus of that consultation (e.g. sports medicine doctor, general practitioner, psychologist or neurologist). In this case, the player presents to a psychiatrist and this likely guides how the consultation will be framed and the attention to emotional, cognitive and behavioural symptoms.

Diagnosis is important to guide treatment and is helpful for player engagement, adherence to a management plan and communicating with other clinicians and professionals who may be involved. For example, sports medicine doctors, when compared to psychiatrists, may be less likely to diagnose a primary mental disorder, consider psychological therapies or prescribe antidepressant medication in those presenting with mood symptoms in the post-concussive period. As with other areas of medicine a multidisciplinary team (MDT) working in a collaborative manner will bring differing perspectives that can be used to develop a holistic treatment and care plan to optimise patient care and outcomes.

The preliminary diagnosis of major depressive disorder as described in ICD-10 (2) would be the most appropriate. B reported a depressed mood persisting most days for at least two weeks. Added to this was a clear history of anhedonia (lack of pleasure in her hobbies) and fatigue. There are additional symptoms of reduced motivation, loss of confidence, irritability, poor sleep and impaired concentration.

Adjustment disorder (2) can be difficult to distinguish from a major depressive episode and there was some overlap in symptomology. There are several recognised subtypes of adjustment disorder depending on the predominant symptoms with the depressive subtypes most likely to be used in this instance. In an adjustment disorder the development of emotional or behavioural symptoms is in direct response to an exceptional and clearly identifiable stressor and/or an obvious change in life circumstance (e.g. divorce) leading to continued unpleasant circumstances. Symptoms begin within three months of a trigger that is considered to be the over-riding causal factor such that symptoms would not have occurred without this. Symptoms are typically mild and transient and resolve within six months. In this case, the origin of her symptoms is thought to be multifactorial and both severe enough and with sufficient associated functional impairment to warrant the diagnosis of a depressive episode.

Persistent post-concussive symptoms should also be considered. Clues to this diagnosis would be symptoms of headache, insomnia, mood changes and fatigue persisting three months after initial injury. The terminology alone is controversial, not universally used and reflects the complexity of underlying pathology and competing perspectives of differing specialties.

Although anxiety symptoms are present they do not predominate and are best seen as a part of another syndrome (a depressive disorder).

Q 2) C, E

The majority of injured athletes recover from concussion within the first month, if not sooner, but physiological recovery is recognised to extend beyond clinical recovery in some athletes (3). Some student athletes report persistent symptoms for many months following head injury, often with varied and non-specific complaints. There can be multiple causes for those symptoms and those individuals are more likely to be included in studies conducted at specialty clinics (4). There is no standard guidance for the assessment of athletes with persistent symptoms that is universally followed. Added to this, there are variations in access to specialist care for players following injury. This is illustrated in the above case study – where the player after initial concussive features had difficulty in identifying which symptoms related to her injury and was therefore not clear whom to approach for assistance.

There are a number of grading systems and assessment tools to assist the clinician in the acute assessment of concussion and its severity. The Concussion in Sport Group through its consensus statements has established the Sports Concussion Assessment Tool (5th edition) (SCAT5) as the recommended tool to support clinical decision-making in the management of head injury (5). The SCAT5 combines previously separate approaches to the assessment of symptoms. Assessment in a consultation includes collection of background information; comprehensive assessment of each symptom (on a scale of none/mild/moderate/severe); cognitive screening (orientation, memory, concentration); and a neurological screen.

Neuropsychological tests also play an important role in the initial management of concussions and in assessing return to sports. In the UK, rugby union uses CogSport in RTP decision-making and an athlete needs to match their baseline CogSport test before contact training is re-introduced (6). This test battery is computerised and ideal for serial assessment. All players at elite-level rugby in the UK will have a pre-season baseline CogSport and SCAT5 every year to contribute to decision-making should there be an injury in the future. When compared to a group of matched non-injured control athletes, concussed athletes display significant deterioration on CogSport measures of psychomotor speed and psychomotor variability (7).

CogSport and SCAT5 have gone some way to assist in understanding the symptomology in this cohort of players and allow standardisation of practice among different sports and professionals.

In professional rugby, where the laws can be consistently applied by expert referees and player skill levels are highest, it might be expected that concussion incidence would decrease with greater awareness of the risk factors in the tackle (8) and the development of tackling techniques to minimise concussion risks. To date, this has not seemed to be the case. More consistent refereeing of high tackles has been promoted by World Rugby (the governing body of rugby union worldwide) in order to attempt to reduce the incidence of concussion (https://laws.worldrugby.org/en/guidelines). Rafferty et al. studied head injuries of professional rugby players over a four-year period (9) and found a lower incidence of match injuries in club rugby compared with international rugby. They also found a statistically significant increased risk of upper limb injuries following concussion when compared to non-concussive injury.

Q 3) C

Planning retirement from elite level sport is not an exact science. Many domestic, social and occupational factors come into play when this significant life event is being considered.

A sports medical doctor or psychiatrist may be asked to assist with the decision, advise on how to negotiate the transition into the 'normal world' or help manage mental health issues that might arise.

It has been suggested that retirement from elite sport and the years that follow are particularly hazardous from a mental health point of view (10). Loss of athletic identity, financial insecurity and lack of secure employment have been hypothesised to contribute. Rugby is one of the many sports to proactively identify this as a time of need for players and to install support. This can occur by way of awareness campaigns, life skills training and employing human resources professionals to help manage the risks and stresses of the transition.

Some perceive rugby players to be heavy users of alcohol with therefore a possibly higher risk of mental health problems and especially those related to alcohol consumption in retirement (11). However, Gouttebarge et al. (12) found that alcohol consumption was not statistically significantly greater in those retiring from the game and found substantially lower levels of alcohol intake in a retired rugby cohort (24%) when compared to those actively playing as measured by the AUDIT-C screening tool. The retired rugby player population also consumed less alcohol when compared with a matched general population and this may be an extension of alcohol restriction and drinking patterns during their professional careers.

The decision to retire after repeated concussive or physical injuries remains complex and there are no evidence-based recommendations to guide the practitioner. In the absence of clear and scientifically valid guidelines, good clinical judgement and common sense remains the mainstay of management. Many non-sporting factors will need to be considered, including age, other financial income possibilities and the wishes of close family members. Performance, injury history and stage of career are also factors.

Concern expressed by the doctor, the patient and other medical or coaching team members is often raised as the prelude to the process of a retirement decision. Far more difficult, and sadly too common, is the trial by media when an athlete with a poor outcome following repeated concussions is reported on with little or no supporting medical evidence and this is then used as the basis for speculation and recommendations about the future of the player concerned.

Q 4)   C

Although epidemiological data is sparse, Gouttebarge et al. have investigated prevalence rates of common mental health symptoms among male rugby players (12) using self-reporting questionnaires. Rates of depression were estimated to be 28% in this cohort and players with these symptoms believed there to be a negative impact on sporting performance. Similar studies have shown higher levels of mental health symptomology in non-contact sports, such as athletics. In other contact sports similar studies have demonstrated a higher prevalence of depressive symptoms with 48% prevalence in Gaelic footballers (13) and 43% in Norwegian soccer players (14). These figures are complicated by low response rates and report symptomology rather than diagnosis data.

Q 5)   False

Player welfare extends to protecting individuals from abuse and there have been recent disclosures of abuse in many sports including rugby union. There is limited literature describing the reasons for this and its longer-term effects. A 'tough masculine' mind-set transcends the sport of rugby union, which may hinder disclosure and result in under-reporting, and the frequency of abuse and resultant dropout rates are difficult to calculate. In common with other sports, rugby union in the UK and Ireland has worked to embrace inclusivity and put safeguards in place to protect participants from harm both on and off the field of play.

Abuse within sporting circles can take many forms. The Rugby Football Union (RFU) aim to create 'a safe and positive environment for everyone to play and enjoy rugby union'. Abuse is defined as a 'violation of an individual's human and civil rights by another person or persons'. The RFU safeguarding policy provides information on the types of abuse and how these might be identified (the policy is available at www.englandrugby.com/govern ance/safeguarding). The policy sets out practical ways of spotting all forms of abuse and frameworks for how these might be addressed, including whistleblowing.

Although precise figures are not available, hazing or team initiations appear to be common in team sports and particularly so in rugby (15). These practices are seen as traditional and a ceremonial 'rite of passage' event usually involving new members of a team. They are usually aimed at forging team bonds and allowing time for players and coaches to get to know each other away from the field of play. However, some have been highlighted in the media and led to court cases and suspensions from the game for players, team management and coaches. The longer-term psychological effects of hazing are unknown at the present time. Hazing often involves college/university teams or individuals of this age and is thought to be more extreme among males. Individuals can be put through ritualistic challenges that involve many types of abuse – physical, psychological and sexual humiliation. Stirling et al. have proposed a list of the psychological consequences of hazing including depression, anxiety and low self-esteem (16). A new player refusing to be initiated will often be punished through social exclusion or even physical abuse. This can be more intense and enduring in its effects than the initiation itself. Thus, hazing is frequently regarded as the lesser of two evils, creating the perception that new players freely choose to be initiated. Hazing initiations therefore become an avenue through which this power structure is maintained and perennially reproduced.

Summary of the Chapter and the Topics Covered

- Atypical presentation of depressive episodes within sport
- End of playing career and transition issues
- The interface and overlap between physical and psychological issues
- Head injury protocols and assessment
- Concussion management and RTP
- Safeguarding player welfare, harassment, abuse and 'hazing' risk within team cultures

References

1. Armstrong LE, VanHeest JL. The unknown mechanism of the overtraining syndrome: Clues from depression and psychoneuroimmunology. *Sports Med.* 2002 [cited 2016 Oct 15];32(3):185–209. Available from: www.ncbi.nlm.nih.gov/pubmed/ 11839081

2. World Health Organization. *International Statistical Classification of Diseases and Related Health Problems – 10th Revision.* World Health Organization. 2011.

3. Kamins J, Bigler E, Covassin T, Henry L, Kemp S, Leddy JJ, et al. What is the physiological time to recovery after

concussion? A systematic review. *Br J Sports Med.* 2017;51(12):935–40.

4. Iverson GL, Gardner AJ, Terry DP, Ponsford JL, Sills AK, Broshek DK, et al. Predictors of clinical recovery from concussion: A systematic review. *Br J Sports Med.* 2017;51: 941–8.

5. Echemendia RJ, Meeuwisse W, McCrory P, Davis GA, Putukian M, Leddy J, et al. The Sport Concussion Assessment Tool 5th Edition (SCAT5). *Br J Sports Med.* 2017 Apr 26 [cited 2019 Dec 1]; bjsports-2017–097506. Available from: http://bjsm.bmj.com/lookup/doi/10.1136/bjsports-2017–097506

6. Yrondi A, Brauge D, LeMen J, Arbus C, Pariente J. Depression et commotions cérébrales dans le sport: une revue de la littérature. *Press Medicale.* 2017;46(10):890–902.

7. Collie A, Maruff P, Makdissi M, McCrory P, McStephen M, Darby D. CogSport: Reliability and correlation with conventional cognitive tests used in postconcussion medical evaluations. *Clin J Sport Med.* 2003;13(1):28–32.

8. Cross MJ, Tucker R, Raftery M, Hester B, Williams S, Stokes KA, et al. Tackling concussion in professional rugby union: A case-control study of tackle-based risk factors and recommendations for primary prevention. *Br J Sports Med.* 2019;53(16):1021–5.

9. Rafferty J, Ranson C, Oatley G, Mostafa M, Mathema P, Crick T, et al. On average, a professional rugby union player is more likely than not to sustain a concussion after 25 matches. *Br J Sports Med.* 2019;53:969-73.

10. Hughes L, Leavey G. Setting the bar: Athletes and vulnerability to mental illness.

Br J Psychiatry. 2012 [cited 2018 Apr 4];200(02):95–6. Available from: www.ncbi.nlm.nih.gov/pubmed/22297587

11. Brown J, Kerkhoffs G, Lambert M, Gouttebarge V. Forced retirement from professional rugby union is associated with symptoms of distress. *Int J Sports Med.* 2017 [cited 2018 Dec 10];38(08):582–7. Available from: www.ncbi.nlm.nih.gov/pubmed/28564743

12. Gouttebarge V, Hopley P, Kerkhoffs GMMJ, Verhagen EALM, Viljoen PW, Lambert M. A 12-month prospective cohort study of symptoms of common mental disorders among professional rugby players. *Eur J Sport Sci.* 2018. Available from: https://doi.org/10.1080/17461391.2018.1466914

13. Gouttebarge V, Tol JL, Kerkhoffs GMMJ. Epidemiology of symptoms of common mental disorders among elite Gaelic athletes: A prospective cohort study. *Phys Sportsmed.* 2016;44(3).

14. Gouttebarge V, Frank B, Aoki H, Kerkhoffs G. Symptoms of common mental disorders in professional football (soccer) across five European countries. *J Sport Sci Med.* 2015;14(4):811–8.

15. Diamond AB, Callahan ST, Chain KF, Solomon GS. Qualitative review of hazing in collegiate and school sports: Consequences from a lack of culture, knowledge and responsiveness. *Br J Sports Med.* 2016; 50:149–53.

16. Stirling AE, Bridges EJ, Cruz EL, Mountjoy ML. Canadian Academy of Sport and Exercise Medicine position paper: Abuse, harassment, and bullying in sport. *Clin J Sport Med.* 2011;21(5):385–91.

Swimming: Adolescent Athlete Training Commitments

Caz Nahman and Carolyn Plateau

Athlete expert advisor: Adrian Moorhouse

Sports psychiatrists specialising in Child and Adolescent Mental Health Services (CAMHS) may encounter younger patients who have exclusively focused on one sport from an early age to the exclusion of other sports and extracurricular activities. Despite regular exercise being linked to better physical and psychological wellbeing, there is an ongoing debate about the appropriate quantity and intensity of training for young athletes to ensure optimal physical and psychosocial development. Young athletes often have to balance educational requirements alongside training demands, navigate changes in their appearance and physique through puberty, and in some cases manage high expectations from coaches and parents. Despite these challenges, most elite junior athletes are unfunded with limited access to sports medicine MDT support. Therefore, a skilled CAMHS psychiatrist needs to explore and factor in such issues with patients in a sensitive and collaborative manner.

Background

EG is a 16-year-old female who had been told by family, friends and coaches throughout her sporting life that she was destined for the Olympics if she kept training hard. She has had many successes to date. She trained with a swimming club since she was aged four. E was a top-three short-distance national swimmer for her age group. Her most recent success was coming 2nd in the under-15 age category at last summer's British championships.

Four years ago, she had moved to an elite training club that has produced several Olympians. She started training before and after school and more recently had significantly altered her diet, increased her training beyond the rigorous programme at her club, and developed obsessive study habits that allowed her little sleep or relaxation time. She had become more anxious at competitions and distressed about her exam results. Although initially she thrived, her swimming performances then started unexpectedly to deteriorate. Her parents and teachers became concerned that she had become more withdrawn and they had been hesitant to share concerns directly with her. Her periods stopped four months ago, and this was the impetus to attend the family doctor to 'go and get things checked over'.

The primary care physician referral letter expressed concerns about her weight loss and amenorrhoeic status. She had a low pulse and blood pressure, slightly abnormal renal function and was referred for further assessment at a paediatric clinic. The referral mentioned lower-than-expected weight, lanugo hair, constipation and cool peripheries and stated 'a previously bright and chatty teenager now seems apathetic, softly spoken and lost her drive'. E denied any difficulties but was referred by the paediatrician to CAMHS with concerns that she possessed suspected disordered eating behaviours.

E was seen by a CAMHS team nurse who took a brief history, did further blood tests and asked for consultant psychiatric input. The notes documented by the consultant CAMHS psychiatrist are outlined below.

Presenting Complaint

'I am just a bit stressed out about my GCSE exam results and accidentally lost a bit of weight, my parents are freaking out ... I have everything under control and really don't need to be here.'

History of Presenting Complaint

During the initial part of the consultation, E exclusively focused on how her swimming performance had deteriorated over the last eight months. She reported that training harder would address this and had made a previous New Year's resolution to do extra training and eat more healthily.

E reluctantly admitted to marked anxiety when around others during swimming competition and training. She had experienced shortness of breath and acute stomach pain, which had even forced her to withdraw mid-competition. She admitted to experiencing a variety of non-specific physical symptoms outside the pool such as 'grumbling tummy' and a band-like headache at the front of her head. She often lay awake at night worrying about what tomorrow might bring and that her parents were going to die (despite showing insight into them being in good health) and was unable to focus on TV programmes. Most of these symptoms had surfaced in the last four months around the time of 'serious revision' for her exams and had steadily worsened until her first exam. E's feelings of 'being on edge' were worse around swimming competition times, even though she was aiming to make the British junior swimming championships, which would take place shortly before she was due to start her A-level studies.

Around a year ago, E recalled making a decision to change her diet and 'really go for it' on the swimming front. This was in response to strong performances and she felt she needed to 'kick on'. E had researched many sports nutrition websites and influencer social media accounts and found advice about 'cleaner, healthier eating', losing body fat and how these would lead to greater performance success. She hinted that she had felt her body shape was not what it should have been 'for a top athlete'. On probing, she admitted that she idolised an Olympic swimmer and thought that their thin, muscular physique was critical to success. Prior to E's healthy eating plan, she was muscular with a BMI of 22. To fuel training, she needed to eat 5–6 times per day, which often included milky drinks and chocolate bars. As a result of her new healthy eating plan, she had swapped processed foods for 'healthier' alternatives and removed sugar, fats and dairy products from her regular diet.

After the initial two months E noticed some weight loss, which did not cause her any undue concern. Her family did not initially notice although her team-mates did and complimented her. E began to weigh herself regularly and began counting her daily calorie consumption. She described feeling guilty when she deviated from her meal plans and was convinced that she would imminently gain weight as a result. E disputed any possible link to her slower performances and instead put this down to her body getting used to a different training regime.

She trained harder and reduced her food intake further. She was sleeping more and felt weak towards the end of races. E's prescribed training programme involved around 40,000 metres of swimming per week. This consisted of two hours of swimming before school 4–5 mornings a week, with an optional additional session from 8.00–8.30am which most athletes did not do. After school there was land (strength and conditioning) training and more two-hour swimming sessions focused on stroke technique, relay work and time trials.

E denied fear of food but admitted that she had been constipated. She maintained that she needed to reduce her weight further. She was pessimistic with regards to the future, felt weak and was uncertain about her future swimming prospects. She denied low mood or thoughts of self-harm.

A former coach met her outside a recent swimming gala and was shocked that E looked pale, possessed thinner hair and was notably less muscular than when she had last seen her over a year ago. These concerns from her former coach prompted her parents to seek professional medical advice.

E's food intake comparing her former diet with her new 'healthier' self-researched plan is outlined in Table 9.1.

Table 9.1 Food diary before and after starting a 'healthy' eating plan.

	Previous Nutritional Plan	**'Healthy Eating Plan'**
5am (before training)	Milky coffee Porridge (made with milk) Raisins and banana	Almond milk coffee Porridge made with water Banana
8.30am (after training)	Peanut butter sandwiches Banana Milky drink	Nothing – no time due to additional optional training
10.30am	Pasta pot at school	Piece of fruit
12.30	Sandwiches Crisps Fruit Small chocolate bar Milky drink	Ryvita with low-fat cheese (no butter or margarine) Green juice Salad
15.00 (before training)	Muffin and milky coffee	Ryvita and cottage cheese
19.30 (after training)	Meat/chicken or fish Potatoes or pasta or rice Vegetables Pudding or ice cream	Smaller portions, no potatoes or pasta Plant-based proteins
Total energy consumed	3880kCal/day	1297kCal/day
Baseline energy needs	**2560–2880** kCals/day	**2560–2880** kCals/day
Energy expenditure doing sport	**1210** kCals/day	**1210** kCals/day
Total energy requirements	**3770–4090** kCals/day	**3770–4090** kCals/day
Summary	Energy requirements for exercise, growth and repair are largely met (+110 to -210kCals/day)	**Current shortfall of 2473 – 2793 kCals/day**

Past Psychiatric History

E had never previously seen a mental health professional or counsellor.

Family History

Her mother disclosed that E's maternal aunt had an 'eating problem' as a teenager and required one inpatient admission.

Past Medical History

E had always been 'healthy' and never needed medical attention. She seldom saw her primary care physician but had occasional physiotherapy for recurrent shoulder strain, which had got worse recently.

Medication

Vitamin D

Multi-vitamin tablet

Social History

E was single and lived with her family in their own home. She had never smoked cigarettes, used alcohol or any illicit medication.

Personal History

E was born at term with no reported birth complications. She was the younger sibling of two and her parents were both from professional, working backgrounds. On review of child-hood developmental milestones, she was reportedly developmentally advanced and very energetic throughout her childhood. She was taken to swimming lessons aged two and a half to see if this might tire her out. She learned to swim very quickly and was able to swim faster than children one to two years older than her. Aged six, she was invited to more regular training with the age eight to nine category group.

At the age of 12 she was invited to a club which had produced teenagers who had competed in world junior championships and senior elite swimmers including several Olympians. E was the youngest swimmer in her group and was soon training twice a day. She appeared to thrive and was top of her year academically alongside her swimming achievements. Her first British championships were as a 14-year-old where she won a bronze medal in the 200m freestyle. By the following year she had improved greatly and had won two gold and one silver medal.

E had never done any other extracurricular sports and swimming had become her sole focus and that of her family. This often resulted in resentment from her older brother who felt she was given too much attention. In fact, her father had reduced his working hours to facilitate her demanding training commitments.

E social contacts were exclusively related to swimming. Unfortunately, this had resulted in E being socially isolated at school, she never attended school parties or social events as her training took up all of her time. She often completed her homework during lunch break because she was training immediately after school. Her peers would tease her stating that she was 'always eating' or 'swotting up at lunchtime'.

Currently, E had been attending a private school and was due to get her GCSE examination results. She had been predicted all 'A' grades and would like to study Biology, Sport Studies and Chemistry for her AS-levels. However, she would like to do this at a new college, as this would give her greater flexibility to commit to her personalised, swimming training. Her parents had voiced their concerns about her intentions although had agreed to re-explore this once she obtained her examination results.

Pre-Morbid Personality

Prior to the significant change in diet, her parents described E as always being a 'bubbly', cheerful character although had now become much more 'serious' and flatter in mood. Her parents reported that she had never been 'fussy' about food and that this was starting to cause a strain within their household.

Forensic History

Nil reported during this consultation.

Collateral History

E's parents had initially been supportive of her dietary changes and expressed guilt for allowing her to choose her own food items during their weekly shop. They hoped that it was just 'a phase' that would settle once she got her exam results. However, they were now of the opinion that her highly restrictive and selective eating habits had become 'too obsessive' and had 'got out of hand'. E insisted that all her food had to be 'vegan, natural, unprocessed and organic'.

This then coincided with her swimming performance deterioration, change in physical appearance ('looked pale and unhappy') and absence of menstruation. When they raised their collective concerns to her, E denied that there was an ongoing issue and she then refused to eat with her family. Furthermore, they disclosed that she had ignored the physiotherapist's advice to rest and had secretly been going on long bike rides 'to maintain fitness'.

Mental State Examination

E was a well-kempt female teenager, who was pale and avoided eye contact. Her speech was reduced in rate and volume and she appeared low in mood. She was orientated in time, place and person. She did not readily discuss her thoughts and tended to deny there were any difficulties. In particular she did not see her reduced and restricted food intake and associated weight loss as a cause for concern; she was fully convinced that these were central to greater sporting success. She was deemed to lack insight on these concerning issues. E normalised her recent strict diet and exercise patterns as simply those of an elite, talented athlete and that she did not want her muscles to disappear. She was dismissive of her parents' expressed concerns and stated she could 'only eat if she had exercised'.

On physical examination, E's body mass index (BMI) was 18.5, which is 90% of median BMI (mBMI) for a 16 year old, her pulse was 42bpm and her blood pressure was low (85/50). The initial blood tests from the primary care physician and paediatric clinic demonstrated sick euthyroid syndrome, hypogonadotrophic hypogonadism and a slightly raised creatinine (see Table 9.2). See Elliot-Sale et al. (1) for a detailed description of endocrine effects of energy deficit in sport.

Table 9.2 Blood test results

Blood test	E's blood test result	Normal range
Hb	145 g/l	120–168
MCV	88 fl	84–102
WCC	3.5 E9/l (low)	4–11 E9/l
Neutrophils	1.8 E9/l (low)	2–7 E9/l
Alkaline phosphatase	32 U/l (low)	40–100 U/l
ALT	40 U/l (above range)	0-33 u/l
Bilirubin	28mmol/l (above range)	0–21mmol/l
TSH	1.1mu/l	0.5–4.2mu/l
fT3	3.9pmol/l (low)	4.7–7.2pmol/l
fT4	10.5pmol/l (low)	10.7–18.4pmol/l
Na+	137mmol/l	134–145mmol/l
K+	3.8mmol/l	3.5–5.3mmol/l
U	1.9mmol/l(low)	2.9–7.5mmol/l
Creatinine	92mmol/l (above range)	48-81mmol/l
B12	1005 (above range)	190-830ng/l
Folate	24 (above range)	3-17microg/l
Vitamin D	24 (low)	<50=insufficiency
FSH	4.6 u/l	Follicular – 1.5 to 11.4 U/l Midcycle: – 3.4–36.2 u/l Luteal: 1.1–9.5 u/l Pregnant: <0.3 u/l
LH	5 u/l	Follicular 0.8–12.5 u/l Midcycle: – 8.7–76.3 u/l Luteal: 0.5–16.9 Pregnant: <1.5
E2	<60pmol/l	Follicular: up to 606pmol/l Midcycle: 253-1930pmol/l Luteal: 121–804
Progesterone	<1 nmol/l	Follicular: 0.5-67 nmol/l Luteal: 7.3–89.1
IGF1	130 microg/l (low)	176–479 microg/l

Risk Assessment

Self: Her menstrual periods had stopped, which is a marker of RED-S. This syndrome has multiple physical and training disadvantages including injury, underperformance and a longer-term risk of poor bone health. She will require tailored, nutritional and physical activity advice to prevent poor bone health, osteoporosis and stress-fracture risk.

E disclosed a one-off episode of self-harm by cutting her forearm when aged 13. She denied any active suicide ideation or intent to end her life.

Others: Nil.

Protective factors: E reported that her relationship with her parents and swimming club friends were strong protective factors.

Case Formulation

E presented as a 16-year-old female junior swimmer who had been competing at national amateur level. She was reported to be an academic 'high achiever' and had been tipped to become a national swimmer who could go on to become an Olympian. From a young age, she specialised in swimming and had limited relationships or identity outside of swimming.

Over the last eight months she had lost weight and there had been a significant deterioration in her swimming performance and physical appearance. She had started to engage in restrictive, eating behaviours and had become fixated on 'healthy eating' trends driven primarily by her desire to succeed in her sport. Despite always feeling tired, she had engaged in higher levels of rigid exercise regimes that were against professional physiotherapy advice.

E possessed a maternal family history of suspected eating disorders (EDs). Along with disordered eating behaviour and exercise addictive behaviour (secondary exercise addiction), there was also clear evidence of anxiety – both in general and specific anxiety around competition.

Plan

- E was initially recommended to reduce her training regime to one session per day and increase her food intake (e.g. drink at least 1 pint per day of whole milk, add in some snacks and put butter back on bread). Following significant prompting by her parents, she agreed to arrange an outpatient appointment with the CAMHS team dietitian to explore meal plan options and alternative high-calorie supplement drinks. She stated she would 'not eat fats' and did not need to put on any weight

- E was provided with a nutrition guidance book specific to competitive adolescent swimmers. It highlighted how swimming requires a considerable energy demand of 400–600kCal/hour and how adequate energy intake (in particular carbohydrate intake) was essential to improve and maintain performance

- E was not prescribed any psychiatric medication following this consultation. She was advised to continue taking her supplement medications given her recent nutritional blood profile. It was reiterated that an adequate dietary intake often corrects nutritional deficiencies without the need for additional supplementation

- As E was not an identified as a purging risk there was no need for advice regarding the electrolyte replacement that is necessary following episodes of self-induced vomiting

- Given her mildly low white cell count and neutrophil blood status, she was advised that she should immediately arrange to see her primary care physician if she experienced any symptoms of infection, e.g. dysuria, productive cough, vomiting or pyrexia. If severely

unwell, she was advised to attend her local accident and emergency department as part of her safety plan
- She was referred to a CAMHS clinical psychologist to determine her suitability for 1:1 psychological interventions. In the interim, she agreed to attend an open group of psychoeducational sessions on the risks of social media with EDs
- It was agreed that at the next outpatient follow up E's swimming coach would attend the consultation too. This would be to provide consensus on E's training regime and whether sanctions should be put in place if she deviated from this plan
- E consented for her treatment information to be shared with her parents and wanted them to be involved with her care plan
- E was provided with educational leaflets and a recommended booklist related to ED recovery. One leaflet advised on where she could access moderated online forums for eating disorder support

Questions

Q 1 What do you think is the most likely diagnosis for E?
   A. Anorexia nervosa
   B. Anxiety disorder
   C. Competition trait anxiety
   D. RED-S
   E. Depression with self-harm

Q 2 Which of the following is not a risk factor for an ED in an athlete?
   A. Personality characteristics (e.g. perfectionism, anxiety, compulsive exercise)
   B. Dieting
   C. Sports-specific requirements (e.g. tight clothing for competition).
   D. Female gender
   E. Parental anxiety

Q 3 Which of the following would be NOT be a valid assessment tool to use in an athlete with a suspected ED? Select all that apply.
   A. The SCOFF questionnaire
   B. A food diary analysed by a nutritionist
   C. BMI or percentage mBMI (%mBMI)
   D. Eating Disorders Examination Questionnaire (EDE-Q)
   E. Compulsive Exercise Test – athlete version

Q 4 What first-line therapy would be most likely to be offered to E, following her diagnosis of an ED?
   A. Family-based treatment/family therapy for anorexia nervosa
   B. CBT for eating disorders (CBT-E)
   C. Adolescent-focused psychotherapy for EDs
   D. Maudsley model of treatment for adults with anorexia nervosa (MANTRA)
   E. DBT

Q 5   Which of the following criteria does an athlete need to meet before returning to training?

A. The athlete should be back to a healthy weight and menstruating

B. Physical health has stabilised; the athlete is able to manage energy intake to maintain restoration and fuel training and is engaged with treatment. A graded return is recommended with reduced training initially

C. A return to sport is not feasible for athletes due to the high relapse risk

D. The athlete should have support in place within the sporting environment from the coaching team

E. The athlete should do yoga and pilates to build strength. A physiotherapist can then decide when they are strong enough to return

Answers

Q 1)   A and possibly B

E's persistent restriction of energy intake, low body weight and intense fear of weight gain are key characteristics of anorexia nervosa in the Diagnostic and Statistical Manual of Mental Disorders, 5th edition, DSM-V (2). Her reluctance to increase her energy intake and her compulsion to exercise in order to 'earn the right' to eat are also indicative. Rigid, obsessive attitudes towards food and the emphasis placed on her body weight and shape are also features. Even though she met the main criteria for RED-S (5) (her energy expenditure exceeds her intake and she is losing weight) it is important not to overlook the underlying psychiatric illness that can manifest as RED-S.

The most recent diagnostic criteria for anorexia nervosa in DSM-V (2) include revisions that are appropriate for athletes, adolescents and males and it is anticipated that the ICD-11 (when released) will be similar. There is now no absolute weight or BMI criterion but rather a description of low weight 'relative to the subjects age, sex, physical health and anticipated developmental trajectory'. Fear of weight gain and/or behaviour which interferes with potential to gain weight and shape and weight concerns are also criteria.

DSM-V differentiates between restricting and purging subtypes of anorexia nervosa. Individuals with the restricting subtype place severe restrictions on the amount and type of food they consume. This might include restricting or avoiding certain food groups, and behaviours such as calorie counting, meal-skipping or rigid rules around food (e.g. only eating foods of a specific colour or food group). Excessive exercise behaviours are also found. A similar restriction of intake can occur in the purging subtype, but individuals also display episodes of binge eating and purging (e.g. self-induced vomiting or use of laxatives).

E was restricting her energy intake, which has led to weight loss and a low body weight for her age. She displayed behaviour that interferes with weight gain and denied the seriousness of her current weight. Young people do not always have the cognitive capacity to give a full account of body image concerns and sometimes this is indirectly surmised from the athlete's presentation. In addition, adolescent BMI can vary significantly with age, with younger adolescents having lower BMIs than adult levels. Best practice recommends that to calculate the degree of a young person's underweight status, the BMI should be expressed as a percentage of the mBMI (6). E's %mBMI was 90%. However, due to being an athlete and having higher muscle mass, %mBMI does not always reflect illness severity.

Many young people who develop anorexia nervosa also present with co-morbid anxiety, which can often precede the ED (3,4). Anxiety and perfectionism are risk factors for developing a restrictive ED and E also experiences anxiety in relation to her swimming and around her exams, as well as some general symptoms.

Q 2) E

EDs are multi-factorial and their development in athlete populations is no different. The prevalence of EDs in athlete populations is significantly elevated (7). Personality character-istics such as perfectionism, rigid thinking and anxiety are common among adolescents with EDs (8) and may be more likely to occur among elite athlete populations. Athletes are expected to be committed to their training, pay close attention to their diet and strive for perfection. The traits required to be a successful athlete are similar to those observed among individuals with an ED (9). Our expectations around what is 'normal' for athletes may make it more difficult to detect potential symptoms of an eating problem. For example, athlete characteristics such as pursuit of excellence, commitment to training and ability to perform through pain can be complicated by overlapping traits of perfectionism, excessive exercise and denial of discomfort as seen in those with an ED.

'Compulsive exercise' refers to rule-driven and rigid exercise behaviours, which may be motivated by weight and shape concerns, or to alleviate negative mood (e.g. anxiety, depressive symptoms). Compulsive exercise attitudes and behaviours have been found commonly to co-occur with EDs, with up to half of all ED patients presenting with unhealthy exercise tendencies (10,11). Compulsive exercise can be predicted by self-critical perfectionism, obsessive-compulsiveness and a drive for thinness in girls (12). Evidence from athlete populations has identified that compulsive exercise increases the risk of eating psychopathology (13,14).

Among males, there may be some differences in the presentation of anorexia nervosa, with preliminary evidence to suggest that muscularity-orientated (as opposed to thin-ness-orientated) disordered eating may be an important phenotype among males with EDs (14). Further research to understand the male experience and presentation of EDs is important.

Q 3) B and C

Food diaries and BMI (or %mBMI) are not sufficient to determine the presence or absence of an ED. The other tools listed are valid screening tools that could help to determine the presence of an ED; it may be appropriate to use one or more of these in initial assessment stages.

The SCOFF questionnaire (16, 17) is a brief screening tool which is often used in primary care to screen for an ED. Answering 'Yes' to two or more questions is indicative of a potential ED. It was originally validated for individuals aged 18–40 years old. The sensitivity is thought to be almost 100% (17), meaning that nearly ALL of true positive cases can be detected with this tool. Recently, Lichtenstien et al. (18) assessed the validity of the SCOFF questionnaire in a Danish adolescent population aged 11–20 and discovered that by changing the number of kg attached to the weight loss criteria to say *any weight loss*, the screening measure could be both sensitive and specific (correctly rule out negative cases).

The EDE-Q (19) has been adopted throughout the UK for monitoring and detecting eating psychopathology. It explores shape and weight concerns, dietary restraint/restriction and preoccupation with, and concern about, eating. A global score is produced, and norms have been developed for adolescents (20). It has also been validated in collegiate athletes (21). As there are some differences in responses by athletes compared to non-athletes (and particularly male athletes) it is suggested to use the EDE-Q alongside other measures too.

Occasionally with a young person (and perhaps more particularly with an athlete) when there is significant denial of an ED, scores on these measures can be below population norms. When this is the case, it can be helpful to use alternative measures with lower face validity for eating psychopathology, but with sufficient sensitivity to detect ED symptoms. For example, the Compulsive Exercise Test assesses compulsive exercise attitudes and behaviours (22,23). An athlete version has been developed and shown to be sensitive in detecting athletes with ED symptoms (scores of 10 or more) (12,13).

Q 4)   A and/or B

As E is still 16 years old, she will be under a CAMHS team. However, those close to 18, depending on consent, capacity and maturity, might be offered a more adult approach (24). Evidence-based treatment for young people with first-onset anorexia nervosa is a family-based approach where parents are supported by therapists to begin to coax their child to eat – initially small amounts 3–6 times per day. The family are encouraged to support the young person to stand up to and take responsibility for the illness. Over time responsibility for managing the illness is gradually handed back to the young person. This approach is thought to result in higher remission rates and more rapid weight gain (25).

Adolescent-focused psychotherapy for anorexia nervosa can be offered as an alternative when weight is not quite so low and where motivation is good. This is an ego-orientated individual therapy and the most promising of individual approaches for young people with anorexia nervosa.

E could also be considered for CBT-E. However, this requires significant insight and a high level of motivation to recover and engage with the treatment process. The rate of progress and weight gain in individual therapeutic approaches is slower than with family-based approaches. Other forms of weight-gain target therapy such as MANTRA have not been studied in patients under the age of 18.

Q 5)   B and D

The IOC consensus statement lists a traffic-light-based system to determine the appropriateness of athlete involvement in both training and competition (5). Concerns over compulsive exercise tendencies or the potential for aspects of the sporting environment to exacerbate the eating problem may also need to be considered prior to any return to sport. A judgement needs to be made that the recovering athlete's mental health is robust enough to avoid significant relapse on returning to sport. This can be facilitated by having strong MDT support to help ensure a smooth transition back into their respective sport.

Acknowledgements

The chapter authors would like to acknowledge support from Lizzie Briasco, MSc, RD, CSSD, Eating Disorder and Sports Dietitian, Chrysalis Centre for Counselling and Eating Disorders, in reviewing the meal plans provided for the case study.

Summary of the Chapter and the Topics Covered

- Adolescent athletes possess unique mental health needs compared to adults
- Adolescent athletes often have less access to sport MDT support
- Treatment in CAMHS may differ from adult biopsychosocial treatment options
- Growth and developmental stages should be factored in during adolescent assessments
- EDs and exercise addiction are often co-morbid (secondary exercise addiction)
- Always rule out an underlying ED in cases of relative energy deficiency in sport (RED-S)
- Parents can play a key role for adolescent athlete consent and treatment issues

References

1. Elliott-Sale K, Tenforde A, Parziale A, Holtzman B, Ackerman K. Endocrine effects of relative energy deficiency in sport. *International Journal of Sport Nutrition and Exercise Metabolism.* 2018;28(4):335–49.

2. American Psychiatric Association. *Diagnostic and Statistical Manual of Mental Disorders*, 5th edition (DSM-5®). Washington, DC. American Psychiatric Publishing. 2013.

3. Godart NT, Flament MF, Lecrubier Y, Jeammet P. Anxiety disorders in anorexia nervosa and bulimia nervosa: Co-morbidity and chronology of appearance. *European Psychiatry.* 2000;15(1:)38–45.

4. Swinburne J, Touyz S. The co-morbidity of eating disorders and anxiety disorders: A review. *European Eating Disorders Review.*2012;15(4):253–74.

5. Mountjoy M, Sundgot-Borgen J, Burke L, Carter S, Constantini N, Lebrun C, et al. The IOC consensus statement: Beyond the female athlete triad – relative energy deficiency in sport. *British Journal of Sports Medicine.*2014;48: 491–97.

6. Le Grange ., Doyle PM, Swanson SA, Ludwig K, Glunz C, Kreipe RE. Calculation of expected body weight in adolescents with eating disorders. *Paediatrics.* 2012;129 (2):438–46.

7. Martinsen M, Sundgot-Borgen J. Higher prevalence of eating disorders among adolescent elite athletes than controls. *Medicine and Science in Sports and Exercise.*2003;45(6):1188–97.

8. Nilsson K, Sundbom E, Hagglof B. A longitudinal study of perfectionism in adolescent onset anorexia nervosa-restricting type. *European Eating Disorders Review.* 2008;16(5):386–94.

9. Thompson RA, Sherman RT. The last word on the 29th Olympiad: Redundant, revealing, remarkable, and redundant. *Eating Disorders: The Journal of Treatment and Prevention.*2009;17:97–102. https://doi .org/10.1080/10640260802570163

10. Monell E, Levallius J, Mantilla EF, Birgegard A. Running on empty – a nationwide large-scale examination of compulsive exercise in eating disorders. *Journal of Eating Disorders.* 2018;6:11.

11. Dalle Grave R, Calugi S, Marchesini G. Compulsive exercise to control shape or weight in eating disorders: Prevalence, associated features and treatment outcome. *Comprehensive Psychiatry.* 2008; 49 (4):346–52.

12. Goodwin H, Haycraft E, and Meyer C. Psychological risk factors for compulsive exercise: A longitudinal investigation of adolescent boys and girls. *Personality and Individual Differences.* 2014 68:83–86.

13. Plateau CR, Shanmugam V, Duckham RL, Goodwin H, Jowett S, Brooke-Wavell KSF, et al. Use of the Compulsive Exercise Test with athletes: Norms and links with eating psychopathology. *Journal of Applied Sport Psychology.* 2014; 26(3):287–301.

14. Plateau CR, Arcelus J, Meyer C. Detecting eating psychopathology in female athletes by asking about exercise: Use of the Compulsive Exercise Test. *European Eating Disorders Review.* 2017;25(6):619–24.

15. Murray SB, Nagata JM, Griffiths S, Calzo JP, Brown TA, Mitchison D, et al. The enigma of male eating disorders: A critical review and synthesis. *Clinical Psychology Review.* 2017;57:1–11.

16. Hill LS, Reid F, Morgan JF, Lacey JH, SCOFF: The development of an eating disorder screening questionnaire. *International Journal of Eating Disorders.* 2010;43(4):344–51.

17. Morgan JF, Reid F, Lacey JH. The SCOFF Questionnaire: A new screening tool for eating disorders. *British Medical Journal.* 1999; 319: 1267–468.

18. Lichtenstein MB, Daugaard-Hemmingsen, S, Storving R. Identification of eating disorder symptoms in Danish adolescent with the SCOFF Questionnaire. *Nordic Journal of Psychiatry.*2017; 71(5):340–47.

19. Fairburn CG, Beglin SJ. Eating Disorder Examination Questionnaire (6.0). In Fairburn CG. *Cognitive Behavior Therapy and Eating Disorders.* New York. Guilford Press. 2008.

20. White HJ, Haycraft E, Goodwin H, Meyer C. Eating disorder examination questionnaire: Factor structure for adolescent girls and boys. *International Journal of Eating Disorders.* 2014;47 (1):99–104.

21. Darcy AM, Hardy KK, Crosby RD, Lock J, Peebles R. Factor structure of the Eating Disorder Examination Questionnaire (EDE-Q) in male and female college athletes. *Body Image.*2013;10(3):399–405.

22. Meyer C, Taranis L, Haycraft E. Compulsive exercise and eating disorders. *European Eating Disorders Review.* 2011;19 (3):174–89.

23. Taranis L, Touyz S, Meyer C. Disordered eating and exercise: Development and preliminary validation of the compulsive exercise test. *European Eating Disorders Review.* 2011;19(3):256–68.

24. Golden NH, Katzman DK, Sawyer SM, Ornstein RM, Rome ES, Garber AK, et al. Update on the medical management of eating disorders in adolescents. *Journal of Adolescent Health.* 2015;56(4):370–75.

25. Lock J, Le Grange D, Agras WS, Moye A, Bryson SW, Jo B. Randomized clinical trial comparing family-based treatment with adolescent-focused individual therapy for adolescents with anorexia nervosa. *Archives of General Psychiatry.* 2010;67 (10):1025–32.

Tennis: Trauma and Tours

Tim Rogers and Jo Larkin

Athlete expert advisor: Naomi Cavaday

Sports psychiatrists often encounter athletes in mental health distress following significant trauma. Early identification can be difficult because athletes may mask trauma-related distress, even though this can negatively impact upon function, performance or injury recovery. Professional tennis differs from other sports because of extensive travel, resource limitations and the emphasis placed upon individual competition. Sensitively demonstrating an understanding of the unique aspects of each high-performance culture, and the effects of trauma upon training and competition, is key to engaging athletes. Those experiencing trauma-related distress require an evidence-based biopsychosocial plan of support.

Background

AB is a 17-year-old English athlete and college student, in the midst of transition into professional tennis. She is academically high-achieving and got straight As in school examinations around three months ago. Following her results she immediately left to compete in an international pro circuit tennis event. While abroad and dining in a restaurant, she and her coach directly witnessed a mass shooting. Two people were killed and others were wounded at the scene. One died from their injuries later. A knew nothing about the reasons for the attack, nor did she know the deceased. She had tended to a neck wound in one injured person, while a crowd of people waited for emergency services to arrive on scene. This victim passed away despite prolonged attempts to resuscitate him.

A acquired minor injuries and decided not to compete in the tournament. She immediately returned home to her parents in the UK, appearing distraught and in a state of shock. Thereafter, she found that she spoke little about what happened. Over the coming weeks, she continued to train. She feared that other pathway athletes would edge ahead of her in their development if she took time out. She noticed early mornings became more difficult. Her ability to endure long matches seemed to diminish. On court, arousal and anger issues arose for which she was not generally known. Pain from a recurrent achilles tendonitis seemed to have flared up.

A gained the courage to confide in her coach that she had hardly slept because of repeated terrible dreams. She made him promise not to tell her parents, which made the coach uncomfortable. Her coach sought the advice of the sports and exercise medicine consultant, who made a referral for an assessment with a consultant sports psychiatrist. The consultation notes from a confidential nearby clinic are below.

Presenting Complaint

'I've been told to come here really. The sports doc thinks I've got post-traumatic stress but I'm not sure whether that applies to me.'

History of Presenting Complaint

Since her first night back in the UK, A has been experiencing traumatic nightmares. These bad dreams have slightly reduced in frequency but have not abated. She estimated that she woke up several times each night. She continued to remember what happened every day, even though she would rather forget. There were no dissociative flashbacks but she did find intrusive memories very upsetting. She recalled how the victim's blood seeped through her fingers and how traumatic memories made her feel cold and slightly shaky. A admitted to avoiding red-coloured items, such as recovery drinks or red branding on her tennis equipment, as this triggered bad memories. She struggled to understand why she remembered this so vividly, because the exact details of what happened were hard to consciously recall.

A reported that watching the news felt different, like an endless stream of violent events. She described often feeling like she could jump out of her skin. Her concentration seemed altered. This had affected her in various ways, including her ability to endure long matches and to complete assignments. A gave herself little time to recover. She had expected that throwing herself back into training would be a good distraction and would help her move on. Furthermore, she did not want to lose her ranking to other players, mindful that there were 'no points without playing'. As a tennis athlete she possessed no employment contract per se. Her income depended heavily upon retaining match time. A described the stress of having to be 'CEO of me' despite her youth and inexperience. This often felt daunting.

Since the shooting, she often felt tight and could not enjoy the feeling of hitting a ball anymore. A particularly struggled with feelings of guilt, believing she should have intervened sooner or that she should have done other things differently. Friends reassured her but this was hard to accept. She admitted feeling extremely guilty after damaging expensive equipment during a recent match, paid for by her sponsor. A agreed that she had become withdrawn and less in control of her emotions. Little things had begun to bother her more than they should. This change in behaviour was commented upon by team-mates.

For many years, A had been intrinsically motivated, with an intense personal drive to become the best version of herself. Both she and her parents had jumped at the opportunity to begin receiving support from her national tennis organisation. Her parents had understood little about what the lifestyle of a professional tennis player might be like. Given this context, she became tearful when admitting that, of late, motivation had become extrinsic. She had only really been playing to avoid her parents' disapproval. Walking on court, competitions felt meaningless compared to someone having lost their life. Tennis had always 'felt like everything'. She had never imagined not playing. 'Tennis athlete' had always been the way she had defined herself. Schoolmates were in awe of exotic trips around the world. The sudden feeling that she might want to choose another path in life – live a different identity – had left her feeling anxious.

Her father had struggled to understand the extent of the effect of the shootings upon her. He had told her to 'push on' and that 'all top players go through things like this'. His view was that this could be done if she 'showed she wasn't mentally weak'. Both of her parents had told her she needed to 'go pro'. They wanted her to consider home-schooling to enable this. A had repeatedly been ruminating about the size of her parents' investment of time and money in her tennis over the years. Travelling and one-to-one coaching costs had been high.

Past Psychiatric History

A had never previously seen a mental health professional or counsellor. She denied any history of childhood mental disorder such as inattention or hyperactivity. She denied ever having felt suicidal in the past or having harmed herself.

She and her parents attended a special workshop to help them deal with the demands of competing but felt dismissive of this. A had sessions with a sport and exercise psychologist who helped her control physiological arousal when serving, spent time reflecting upon team values but never individually explored feelings away from the court.

Family History

There was no formally diagnosed family history of mental disorder.

Past Medical History

Current left foot achilles tendonitis (seeing a physiotherapist)

History of 'tennis leg' (gastrocnemius injury)

Menarche aged 12

Medication

Ibuprofen 400mg PRN

Social History

A was single, heterosexual in orientation and lived in her family home. She had never been in a significant intimate relationship before. There was no history of problem drinking, gambling, doping violations or use of other banned performance enhancements.

After checking whether she could speak in confidence, she admitted trying a line of cocaine powder at a friend's address but was unable to confirm exactly how much. She had not confided in anyone else about it. She did it 'not to feel' anymore. She believed she had probably evaded detection but worried for days that she had thrown away everything she had worked for. Her reflection was of shock that she had found herself in the position of riding her luck in this manner.

Personal History

A was born in New York State, USA, with no reported problems with gestation or delivery. She attained all expected childhood developmental milestones and avoided any significant ill health in childhood. At the age of five she moved from America to the UK with her family and attended a private UK primary school. This was after the 2007 financial crisis and her American father needed to find a new investment-banking role. Her mother was a lawyer who retired when it became clear that one or more of their children might have the opportunity to play sport professionally. Her mother played National Collegiate Athletic Association tennis growing up but never turned professional.

A denied any history of personal abuse (bullying, physical, emotional or sexual). She mostly had a good relationship with her siblings, although she described falling out when making comparisons of each others' achievements. She recalled a couple of incidents of domestic abuse between her parents, who often argued in front of her. She wondered whether they had only stayed together for her and the siblings.

Following the successful completion of 11+ entrance exams she gained a place at a selective grammar school. She described always having had a healthy network of friends and being above average with her academic achievements. A's journey into tennis began with summer camps aged five. Her parents stopped her playing recreational netball quite early, so that she could focus on tennis. A was keen to remain in college so that she could retain 'normal' social connections outside tennis. By the age of 16, she had attained the number one singles ranking in her age group and was selected onto a national funding programme scheme for gifted players. This trajectory was unexpected because she was ranked significantly lower during earlier years. Dealing with the pressure of 'suddenly being top' was challenging and, at times, she noticed fears around both success and losing.

A's parents shared a belief in 'tough love' and neither were particularly warm in parenting style. She tended not to confide in them when in a difficult moment. By way of example she recalled that as a child, when she lost a match, she would often go and sit alone behind the back fence. Her family would tend to leave her to gather her thoughts there. Car journeys home would tend to be tense. Her parents had sometimes decided not to speak to her (or even to punish her with extra training) if they felt she had not performed on court. A felt as though it was much less of a struggle to get her father, in particular, to be forthcoming with praise when things went well: 'a good result would get talked about all weekend but, if it went the other way, you didn't want to be around him'. She had overheard her father boasting to friends and colleagues about her achievements.

A had been fortunate to avoid serious injury. Her ability to transition through serious challenges had not previously been tested.

Pre-Morbid Personality

Prior to the shooting, A believed her friends would have described her as the 'joker' even though, deep down, she was reflective and a deep thinker. She was aware of not normally being someone to talk openly about how she felt. She described the sense of parental approval being contingent upon tennis achievements. A reflected upon the way in which this had both long felt stressful and had also fostered her innate perfectionism. She recognised a sense of satisfaction from intense effort in training but also the setting of excessively high standards for herself at times. This had led to ruminating over mistakes and a tendency towards unhealthy self-criticism. In the past, she had occasionally resorted to unhealthy coping strategies such as the use of feigned injury or illness to avoid punishment or competing.

Forensic History

Nil. No cautions or convictions. Never previously arrested.

Collateral History

She did not wish her coach or parents to be contacted for further information.

Mental State Examination

A presented as a 17-year-old Caucasian female who was well-kempt and pleasant in interaction. She was wearing her official tennis training kit and had a left-sided antalgic gait. She was guarded initially and eye contact improved as the consultation progressed. Noted to be tearful when she discussed how she was no longer enjoying tennis. She was not objectively hypervigilant. Her speech was quiet but otherwise unremarkable in rate, tone and quality. Her subjective and objective mood was flat but reactive.

She described re-experiencing intrusive and distressing memories of the victim's blood associated with feeling cold and, sometimes, slightly shaky. She had started to avoid red-coloured items. She possessed recurrent graphic and vivid nightmares and became easily startled ('jump out of my skin'). Her thoughts were focused on guilt about a shooting victim and how she could and should have done more to help him. She reported difficulty concentrating while playing extended tennis matches and felt less positive about her future career. A disclosed that she did not want to attend the assessment, 'if my parents found out that I saw a shrink they would think I've become weak and attention-seeking'. There was no evidence of psychomotor retardation, thought disorder or dissociation.

A presented with relatively good insight into her change in character. Disinterest in tennis was reflected through a switch to extrinsic motivation for competing. She was aware that there had been an impact upon her daily function and mood. She did not believe that she needed any treatment or psychiatric follow up, 'all of this is pretty normal given what I've been through'. She presented mainly because both her coach and the chief medical officer said it was 'important'. She was fully orientated in time, place and person although still possessed some 'patchy' memory gaps regarding the incident.

She consented for key assessment findings to be shared with relevant members of her sport multidisciplinary team (sMDT). She had to be reassured that she would not be 'dropped' from the performance programme and demonstrated mental capacity to consent to information sharing.

Risk Assessment

Self: There was no evidence of thoughts about self-harm or suicide, nor any intention or plan in this respect. Likely some degree of worsening ankle injury risk if she continued to play with ongoing psychological changes. No previous history of self-harm

To others: No evidence of this

From others: Potential risk of disengagement from professional support and intervention due not just to personal beliefs about her symptoms being 'normal considering' but also because of her parents' expressed attitudes about needing to 'push on' and 'not be mentally weak'

Protective factors: A was surrounded by a concerned multidisciplinary team of sports professionals in addition to the assessing sports psychiatrist, including a sports and exercise medicine consultant, her physiotherapist, her strength and conditioning trainer and her tennis coach, who had also sought support for the same incident

Case Formulation

A presented as a 17-year-old female college student and junior tennis player close to competing in professional tennis. She and her coach experienced an unexpected trauma around three months ago while competing abroad, rapidly resulting in a severe presentation of PTSD.

There was no family history of mental health illness. Pre-trauma predictors in this case included cognitive styles (unhealthy perfectionism, compartmentalisation), issues around pre-trauma psychological resilience that related to the athlete's support network and family system (adverse childhood experiences, threat of income and ranking loss and her parents' attitudes to achievement and success). These issues may also have a role in the maintenance of the disorder.

A was delayed in seeking help for various reasons including unhealthy attitudes towards showing weakness and her own fears about who among the younger players might overtake her ranking if she were unable to compete. There were protective factors within her sMDT setup.

Plan

- Sought consent to confidentially share key pieces of information with the sMDT. Benefits of this in terms of joined-up working and the management of risk explained. Reassurance needed that this would not lead to removal from the performance programme
- Explored myths about 'strength', 'weakness' and mental health together with the athlete to engage her in a plan for wellbeing and recovery
- Joint sessions offered to include the athlete's parents. The sMDT discussed together the prevailing coaching team dynamics in making an assessment of whether a psychologically safe environment existed for this athlete
- Local guidelines around safe sport, duty of care and safeguarding considered and followed, in this case in relation to the monitoring of ongoing emotional abuse risk
- Agreed not to offer drug treatments for the treatment of PTSD in the first instance, both due to the athlete's age and her preference
- Athlete referred for a trauma-focused CBT intervention delivered by a chartered clinical psychologist experienced of working in high-performance sporting environments
- The option of a later *group* trauma-focused CBT intervention to include the athlete's coach was kept in mind, because there had been an event leading to their shared trauma
- These interventions included:
  - psycho-education about reactions to trauma; strategies for managing arousal
  - safety planning
  - elaboration and processing of the trauma memories
  - restructuring trauma-related meanings for the individual
  - help to overcome avoidance behaviours
  - graded exposure to red objects and colour
- Symptom and functional level monitored over time by the sports psychiatrist. In this case it was not necessary to reconsider SSRI antidepressant medication
- Athlete's coaching team were: advised about an expected RTP schedule; advised about how best to support A when once more competing
- An appropriate safety plan was prepared including agreement about when and how to contact the sports psychiatrist again if needed

Questions

Q 1 Which of the following is a self-report measure of International Classification of Diseases (ICD-11) (1) PTSD and complex PTSD?
A. Trauma screening questionnaire
B. Startle, physically upset by reminders, anger and numbness self-report screen (SPAN)
C. Primary care PTSD screen
D. The International Trauma Questionnaire (ITQ)
E. Short Post-Traumatic Stress Disorder Rating Interview (SPRINT)

Q 2 Psychological disorders resulting from trauma will present:
A. Within 6 months of the index event
B. At least within 6 to 12 months
C. Not longer than 1 to 5 years afterwards
D. Not longer than 5 to 10 years afterwards
E. At any point in time afterwards

Q 3 The National Institute for Health and Care Excellence (NICE) NG116 guideline (12) post-traumatic stress disorder evidence review identified *no* evidence for which of the following biopsychosocial treatment intervention options?
A. Trauma-focused CBT
B. Self-help
C. Psychologically focused debriefing
D. Eye movement desensitisation and reprocessing (EMDR)
E. Non-trauma-focused CBT interventions targeted at specific symptoms

Q 4 Franck (13) studied athletes' adjustment patterns in the junior-to-senior transition. Which of the following were *not* found to be a characteristic relevant for both progressive and sustainable adjustment patterns?
A. Keeping a primary focus on sport (but also having attention to other spheres of life)
B. Having attention to other spheres of life (outside of sport)
C. High athletic identity
D. Financial support and sponsorship
E. Motivation to reach senior level

Q 5 According to a study by Leahy et al. (17), elite athletes reported that their rates of reported sexual abuse perpetrated by sports personnel were approximately 25% higher in comparison to club-level athletes. True or false?

Answers

Q 1) D

Although all of the above are validated trauma measures, the ITQ was developed to be consistent with the organising principles of the ICD-11, as set forth by the WHO. These

Below are a number of problems that people sometimes report in response to traumatic or stressful life events. Please read each item carefully, then circle one of the numbers to the right to indicate how much you have been bothered by that problem in the past month.

	Not at all	A little bit	Moderately	Quite a bit	Extremely
P1. Having upsetting dreams that replay that part of the experience or clearly related to the experience?	0	1	2	3	4
P2. Having powerful images or memories that sometimes come into your mind in which you feel the experience is happening again in the here and now?	0	1	2	3	4
P3. Avoiding internal reminders of the experience (for example, thoughts, feelings, or physical sensations)?	0	1	2	3	4
P4. Avoiding external reminders of the experience (for example people, places. conversations, objects, activities or situations)?	0	1	2	3	4
P5. Being 'super-alert', watchful or on guard?	0	1	2	3	4
P6. Feeling jumpy or easily startled?	0	1	2	3	4
In the past month have the above problems:					
P7. Affected your relationships or social life?	0	1	2	3	4
P8. Affected your work or ability to work?	0	1	2	3	4
P9. Affected any other important part of your life such as parenting or school or college work or other important activities?	0	1	2	3	4

Figure 10.1. A copy of the International Trauma Questionnaire (PTSD scoring section)

principles maximise clinical utility and ensure international applicability through a focus on the core symptoms of a given disorder. The ITQ (2) instrument is a brief, simply worded measure, focusing only on the core features of PTSD and complex PTSD (CPTSD), and employs straightforward diagnostic rules. The ITQ (Figure 10.1) is freely available in the public domain to all interested parties: www.traumameasuresglobal.com/itq.

In relation to A, her ITQ results relating to the above were as follows:

- Sum of Likert scores for P1 and P2 = 7 (Re-experiencing in the here and now score – Re)
- Sum of Likert scores for P3 and P4 = 6 (Avoidance score – Av)
- Sum of Likert scores for P5 and P6 = 5 (Sense of current threat – Th)

Completing an ITQ produces results compatible with ICD-11 PTSD because her score (Sum of Re, Av and Th) = 18. A diagnosis of PTSD requires the endorsement of one of two symptoms from the symptom clusters of (1) re-experiencing in the here and now, (2) avoidance and (3) sense of current threat, plus endorsement of at least one indicator of functional impairment associated with these symptoms. Endorsement of a symptom or functional impairment item is defined as a score > 2. As P8 = 3 (at least one of P7, P8 or P9 > 2) she also meets criteria for PTSD functional impairment.

It is found that 13% of nationally ranked athletes (3) meet criteria for PTSD, with rates up to 25% in performance dancers. It is important to be aware of this possibility, particularly in females. Many different kinds of trauma can lead to PTSD, whether serious accidents, physical or sexual assault, childhood or domestic abuse, exposure to traumatic events at work, serious health problems such as being admitted to intensive care, childbirth experiences such as losing a baby, war, conflict and torture. The shooting in this case is, therefore, a less common cause but it is something that professional tennis players have encountered in the modern era.

In elite sport, the health problem most frequently associated with elevated levels of PTSD symptomatology (specifically hyperarousal symptoms) is the presence of injury (4). Self-efficacy beliefs may impact how an athlete manages the stress of injury. Younger athletes, female athletes and those who have a strong athletic identity may experience greater emotional trauma following injury (5). Traumatic injuries may pose an even greater risk of progression to a chronic trauma-related disorder such as PTSD among athletes who entered their sport with pre-existing trauma exposures (6).

Q 2) E

ICD-11 distinguishes between PTSD and chronic PTSD. The latter differs in presentation and the diagnosis recognises longer-term changes after trauma including disturbances in self-organisation clusters: (1) affective dysregulation, (2) negative self-concept and (3) disturbances in relationships.

Elite athletes commonly develop coping strategies that can be adaptive in the setting of trauma, but may also mask trauma-related symptoms, making trauma-related disorders more difficult to detect. Recent years have seen increased professional and academic focus upon identifying and prioritising mental health in elite athletes (7). Despite this, PTSD may be concealed and challenging to diagnose in this population, who often believe they should be 'mentally tough' through difficult moments or feel additional stigma about admitting to emotional distress (8). Athletes frequently display traits of perfectionism that can also affect whether they are willing to be seen to manifest diminished mental wellbeing without being subject to criticism (9). Early identification of athletes suffering from acute trauma-related symptoms is key because of the finding that early-prolonged exposure and cognitive therapy accelerates recovery (10). Association of Tennis Professionals and Women's Tennis Association athletes often travel relentlessly and can describe a sense of 'being constantly on the road', away from home and sources of support. Routine mental health screening and wider awareness programmes can therefore be more difficult to deliver in the sport of professional tennis because of organisational structures based primarily around individuals and small teams that are transitory. PTSD can significantly impair life functioning and performance on court (11).

The reflection of Naomi Cavaday, former British professional number three tennis player, was that:

> This case study shows how easily mental illness can be seen as a mental weakness in the world of elite sport, not only by parents and coaches but by the players themselves too. We can clearly see how losing the desire to play at a high level is an unexpected consequence of PTSD: causing confusion; causing the player and his parents to read the situation as something he 'just needed to push through' in order to get to the top. It is incredibly difficult for people to work out, in real life, which behaviours are symptoms of a mental illness and which might be the situations that an athlete needs to push through. It is so important for players, parents and coaches to seek advice from a professional in this area and also to feel ok about doing that.

Q 3) C

NICE describes the considerable evidence for trauma-focused CBT, EMDR, self-help and non-trauma-focused CBT interventions targeted at specific symptoms. No evidence was identified for psychologically focused debriefing (for treatment of PTSD symptoms more than one month after trauma) or for human givens therapy. The human givens approach, for reference, theorises that a human being will be emotionally and mentally healthy when essential emotional needs are met and innate mental resources used correctly. NICE did find limited evidence for problem-solving or attention-bias modification, metacognitive therapy, somatic experiencing, reconsolidation of traumatic memories intervention, single-session behavioural therapy, hypnotherapy, psychodynamic therapy, IPT, resilience-oriented treatment, cognitive-behavioural conjoint therapy, family therapy and child-parent psychotherapy using play.

The limited evidence about the use of drug treatments to treat PTSD in young people shows no significant benefits so this was not offered to A. This decision followed guidance from the December 2018 NICE guideline committee (12), relating to drug treatments for children and young people. It should be noted that this finding does *not* apply to the treatment of adults.

Q 4) D

Franck et al. (13) identified adjustment patterns in the junior-to-senior transition based on athletes' dynamics of adjustment during a two-and-a-half-year period, and described the athletes' demographic, personal and transitional characteristics related to the different adjustment patterns. Three profiles were identified with different patterns: a progressive adjustment pattern, a regressive adjustment pattern and a sustainable adjustment pattern. The descriptive statistics indicated that there were differences (with variation in magnitude) between the three profiles at the first measurement in terms of how athletes perceived different transitional characteristics.

Elite junior tennis athletes are often pushed towards winning and talent development by heavily involved parents. This can negatively affect parent–child relationships in which many conflicts between them remained unresolved in later life (14). Such aspects of early environment can confer vulnerability to PTSD. It is found that 'pre-trauma predictors' can include cognitive styles, coping styles and absent traits of psychological resilience (15). In elite athletes, such styles are reviewed by Aron (16) and may include compartmentalisation (learning to subconsciously place simultaneous experiences in separate psychological spaces), dissociation (a psychological mechanisms setting the traumatic memory apart from consciousness) and unhealthy perfectionism (which may manifest as unrealistic personal standards).

Q 5) False

The study found that this was higher still: 46.4% of elite athletes reporting sexual trauma had been abused by sports personnel, compared with 25.6% of the club-level athletes. This is an increase of more than 80%. There are many possible explanations for increased prevalence of PTSD in athletes, whether as a result of increased risk of serious injury (4), concussion (18) or pre-existing trauma exposure (6) through abusive dynamics or experiences within sports teams (17).

Safeguarding is a key consideration in the coach–athlete relationship. Tennis clubs, national associations and countries will each have differing policy and legal frameworks around safeguarding but, in general, the key message is about acting upon concerns in a sensitive but timely way having sought relevant information about the appropriate available support.

Young people engaging in sport should find it fun, confidence building and rewarding. Unfortunately, there have been increased media reports of abuse of positions of trust within sport. Sport personnel working within youth sport often hold positions of trust and authority.

Within the sport setting, athletes aged 16–17 are considered to be particularly vulnerable to sexual abuse and exploitation, even though they can legally consent. This is due to the significant power differential between a coach and a vulnerable, younger athlete. For example, athletes can be highly dependent on their coach, mentor or other adults for their sporting development, success or position within a team. Therefore, any romantic or sexual relationship between a coach and young player is a criminal offence and a breach of code of conduct.

According to the National Society for the Prevention of Cruelty to Children Child Protection in Sport Unit (19), any abuse of a position of trust suspicions should be immediately reported to an organisation's welfare or designated safeguarding lead. Safeguarding in sport is the process of protecting children and adults from harm by providing them a safe space to engage in activity. Everyone working in sport should be familiar with his or her organisation's latest safeguarding protocol.

Within the UK, concerned parties can seek advice from a 24-hour telephone help line: 0808 800 5000.

Summary of the Chapter and the Topics Covered

- The psychiatric sequelae and management of acute trauma through to PTSD, including the atypical presentations within elite sport
- Working as a sport multidisciplinary team (sMDT)
- Organisational and personal stressors faced by individuals within professional tennis
- Athletes' adjustment patterns in the junior-to-senior transition
- Parents and the influence of the family system in junior tennis players' development
- Relationship between injuries and mental illness

References

1. World Health Organization. *International Classification of Diseases 11th Revision*. 2019. Available from: https://icd.who.int/en/

2. Hyland P, Shevlin M, Brewin CR, Cloitre M, Downes AJ, Jumbe S, et al. Validation of post-traumatic stress disorder (PTSD) and complex PTSD using the International Trauma Questionnaire. *Acta Psychiatr Scand*. 2017;136:1–10.

3. Thomson P, Jaque SV. Visiting the muses: Creativity, coping, and PTSD in talented dancers and athletes. *American Journal of Play*. 2016;8:363–78.

4. Bateman A, Morgan KD. The postinjury psychological sequelae of high-level Jamaican athletes: Exploration of a posttraumatic stress disorder–self-efficacy conceptualization. *Journal of Sport Rehabilitation*. 2019;28(2):144–52.

5. Padaki AS, Noticewala MS, Levine WN, Ahmad CS, Popkin MK, Popkin CA. Prevalence of posttraumatic stress disorder symptoms among young athletes after anterior cruciate ligament rupture. *OrthopJ Sports Med*. 2018;6(7). DOI:10.1177/2325967118787159.

6. Cloitre M, Stolbach BC, Herman JL, van der Kolk B, Pynoos R, Wang J, et al.

A developmental approach to complex PTSD: Childhood and adult cumulative trauma as predictors of symptom complexity. *Journal of Traumatic Stress.* 2009;22:399–408.

7. Reardon CL, Hainline B, Aron CM, Baron D, Baum AL, Bindra A, et al. Mental health in elite athletes: International Olympic Committee consensus statement (2019). *Br J Sports Med.* 2019;53 (11):667–99.

8. Bauman NJ. The stigma of mental health in athletes: Are mental toughness and mental health seen as contradictory in elite sport? *Br J Sports Med.* 2016;50:135–6.

9. Chen LH, Kee YH, Tsai YM. An examination of the dual model of perfectionism and adolescent athlete burnout: A short-term longitudinal research. *Social Indicators Research.* 2009;91:189–201.

10. Wenzel T, Zhu LJ. Posttraumatic stress in athletes. In: Baron DA, Reardon C, Baron SH, eds. *Clinical Sports Psychiatry: An International Perspective.* New York. Wiley. 2013. p.102–14.

11. Shalev AY, Ankri Y, Gilad M, Israeli-Shalev Y, Adessky R, Qian M, et al. Long-term outcome of early interventions to prevent posttraumatic stress disorder. *J Clin Psychiatry.* 2016;77 (5):e580–e587.

12. The National Institute for Health and Care Excellence. *Post-Traumatic Stress Disorder Guideline* [NG116]. 2018. Available from: www.nice.org.uk/guidance/ng116/chapter/ Recommendations#management-of-ptsd- in-children-young-people-and-adults

13. Franck A, Stambulova NB, Ivarsson, A. Swedish athletes' adjustment patterns in the junior-to-senior transition. *International Journal of Sport and Exercise Psychology.* 2018;16(4):398–414.

14. Lauer L, Gould D, Roman N, Pierce M. How parents influence junior tennis players' development: Qualitative narratives. *Journal of Clinical Sport Psychology.* 2010;4(1):69–92.

15. Wild J, Smith KV, Thompson E, Béar F, Lommen MJJ, Ehlers A. A prospective study of pre-trauma risk factors for post-traumatic stress disorder and depression. *Psychol Med.* 2016;46 (12):2571–82.

16. Aron CM, Harvey S, Hainline B, Hitchcock ME, Reardon CL. Post-traumatic stress disorder (PTSD) and other trauma-related mental disorders in elite athletes: A narrative review. *Br J Sports Med.* 2019; 53:779–84.

17. Leahy T, Pretty G, Tenenbaum G. A contextualized investigation of traumatic correlates of childhood sexual abuse in Australian athletes. *International Journal of Sport and Exercise Psychology.* 2008;6:366–84.

18. Brassil HE, Salvatore AP. The frequency of post-traumatic stress disorder symptoms in athletes with and without sports related concussion. *Clinical and Translational Medicine.* 2018;7:25.

19. Sport England. *Our Work; Safeguarding.* Available from: www.sportengland.org /our-work/safeguarding/

Appendix: International Society for Sports Psychiatry Curriculum 2018

By completing this book we have aimed to cover the International Society for Sports Psychiatry curriculum (2018) and to provide an overview of the emerging field of sports psychiatry. Topics covered include:

- Anxiety in athletes
- Attention deficit hyperactivity disorder in athletes
- Barriers to athletes accessing mental health resources
- Bipolar disorder in athletes
- Child and adolescent sports psychiatry
- Concussion and mental health symptoms in athletes
- Culture in sports
- Depression in athletes
- Eating disorders and other body image disorders in athletes
- Ethical issues in sport
- Exercise addiction
- Exercise as a treatment for mental illness
- Gambling disorder in athletes
- Harassment and abuse (non-accidental violence) in sport
- Medication use for psychiatric disorders in athletes
- Overtraining syndrome
- Post-traumatic stress disorder and other trauma-related disorders in athletes
- Psychotherapy for psychiatric disorders in athletes
- Relationship between injuries and mental illness
- Retirement in athletes
- Sleep in athletes
- Substance use disorders in athletes
- Suicide risk in athletes

Index